ALTERNATIVE ANSWERS TO

PAIN

ALTERNATIVE ANSWERS TO
PAIN

RICHARD THOMAS

CONSULTANT
≡People's Medical Society.

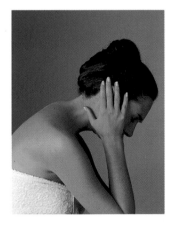

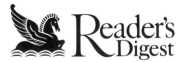

The Reader's Digest Association, Inc.

Pleasantville, New York • Montreal

A Reader's Digest Book
Conceived, edited, and designed by
Marshall Editions Ltd.
The Orangery
161 New Bond Street
London W1Y 9PA

Library of Congress Cataloging in Publication
Data
Thomas, Richard, 1943-
  Pain/ Richard Thomas : consultant People's
Medical Society.
      p. cm. -- (Alternative Answers to)
   ISBN 0-7621-0245-4
   1. Pain 2. Pain--Alternative treatment. I. Title.
II. Series.
RB127.T497 2000
616'.0472—dc21   99-29962

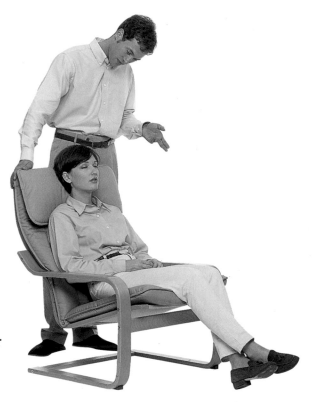

EDITORS	Clare Hill, Richard Shaw, Sue Harper
DESIGNER	Sue Storey
ART EDITOR	Frances deRees
MANAGING EDITOR	Anne Yelland
MANAGING ART EDITOR	Patrick Carpenter
EDITORIAL DIRECTOR	Ellen Dupont
PICTURE RESEARCH	Elaine Willis
EDITORIAL COORDINATOR	Rebecca Clunes
EDITORIAL ASSISTANT	Sophie Sandy
INDEXER	Laura Hicks
PRODUCTION	Nikki Ingram
COVER PHOTOGRAPH	Tony Latham

Originated by PICA Colour Separation Pte
Printed and bound in Italy by New Interlitho Spa

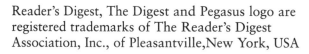

The information and
recommendations given in this book
are not intended to be a substitute
for medical advice. Consult your
doctor before acting on any of the
suggestions in this book. The author
and publisher disclaim any liability,
loss, injury, or damage incurred as a
consequence, directly or indirectly, of
the use and application of the
contents of this book.

Contents

Introduction

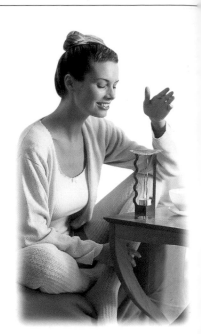

There are many ways, both conventional and complementary, of alleviating pain. Conventional medicine has been successful in treating pain of many different origins—acute, or short term pain, and chronic pain that persists for weeks, months or even years. Conventional medicine—which can often take the form of prescription drugs—has its drawbacks, however. Many people are concerned about taking often powerful medication for long periods of time. And, while drugs may relieve pain, they may not tackle the cause of the pain.

Conventional doctors – along with their patients —are increasingly receptive to complementary therapies. Osteopathy and chiropractic, nutritional and dietary therapy and acupuncture, for example, are among therapies once considered complementary that are increasingly offered in conventional hospitals; reflexology and aromatherapy are commonly practiced in hospice units. Such therapies can be helpful in relieving pain. This book introduces therapies that many people have found useful in treating pain. Some involve no more than simple lifestyle changes: losing some weight may help some people, and paying attention to the quality of the food you eat, including lots of fresh fruit and vegetables, and whole grains, will boost your overall health. Others involve more active participation. They include movement therapies such as t'ai chi and yoga, which have proven successful in relieving pain which has its origin in tension or stress. Such therapies are simple to learn from a practitioner and can then be practiced at home on your own. Also helpful in relieving pain are "hands-on" therapies such as massage, reflexology, and shiatsu.

The basic premise of many complementary therapies is that they are holistic, treating the whole person, mind, body and spirit, rather than treating a collection of symptoms. If you consult a homeopath or herbalist, for example, he or she will focus on you as a person, rather than asking specifically about your pain, although relieving your pain will be a part of any treatment suggested.

When we are tired or worried, pain seems more severe. Those who can relax are often better able to handle pain than those who cannot. For this reason many of the therapies in this book are concerned with the power of the mind. Meditation, relaxation, biofeedback and hypnosis can all help to alleviate pain, or to make you better able to cope with your pain. If you have never tried a complementary therapy, one of the relaxation therapies may be the ideal place to start.

Warning: Whatever its origin, it is vital to identify the cause of your pain. It is essential to seek an expert diagnosis of what is wrong before you decide whether the therapies suggested in this book may be helpful for you. Do not attempt self diagnosis: many apparently minor problems can be symptoms of more serious illness. Even if you feel your conventional doctor can offer no further help, keep him or her informed about any therapy you intend to try and do not cut down on your conventional medication without his or her agreement. With some conditions, such as asthma, cutting down on conventional medication can be life-threatening.

How to use this book

This book works in several ways. You can read it from the beginning to the end to understand the ways in which pain affects your body and to discover your treatment options. But you can also browse through it, using the "Find out more" suggestions as your guide, to learn all about a specific condition and its treatment. Or you could dip into the treatments and therapies chapter to explore all your options in overcoming pain, or learning to live with it.

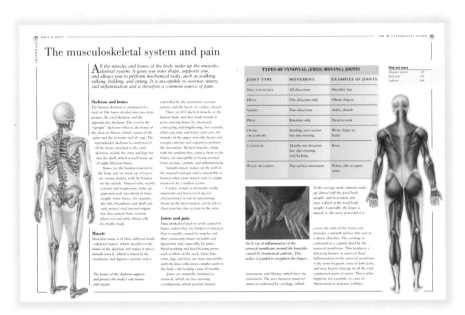

1 *Chapter one explains what pain is, and why we feel pain. It also looks at how pain affects the body's major systems: the musculoskeletal, nervous, digestive, and urinary systems.*

2 *Chapter two explains the many ways in which pain can be treated, both conventional and complementary. In each case the philosophy underpinning the therapy is explained and the ways in which it may help to relieve pain are detailed.*

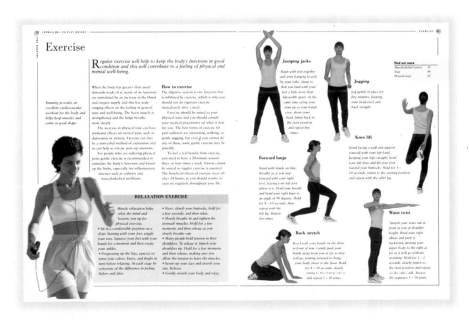

3 *Chapter three offers practical remedies that are easy to use at home to treat every type of pain. Organized by the part of the body involved, this chapter lists specific therapies that may benefit pain sufferers, details dosages where appropriate, and offers advice on when practitioner-administered therapies may be useful.*

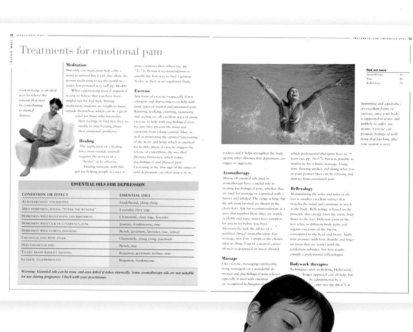

Pain is an individual phenomenon; each person may feel it differently. As a result, a therapy that relieves one type of pain in one person, may not be effective in treating the same pain in another. The three chapters of this book, taken together, offer a comprehensive guide to the causes, treatment, and relief of pain.

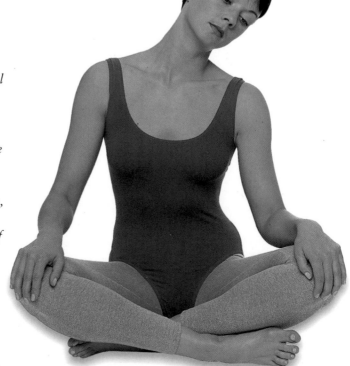

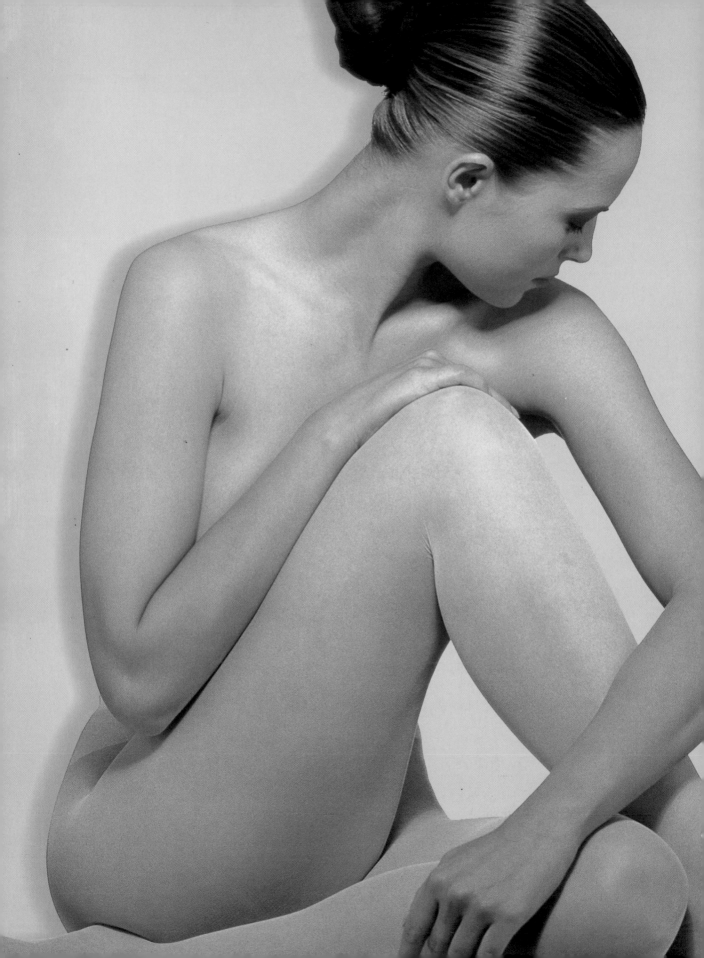

1
WHAT IS

PAIN?

There are two basic types of pain. Acute pain is a normal bodily response to injury or illness, and is usually short-lived. Chronic, or long-term, pain is often a result of chronic disease or previous injury or surgery and results from the way we heal.

No two people experience pain in exactly the same way. One of the worst things about pain is that, although real, it is elusive and very individual and is therefore difficult to describe to other people. This makes finding the cause of the pain and getting help more difficult.

This chapter attempts to define pain, explains why we feel pain, and describes how pain affects the body's systems.

Naming pain

The word "pain" is usually used to describe a wide range of physical effects, but is best defined as a sensory or emotional response to actual or impending tissue damage. Emotional distress makes as many demands as physical pain. Pain can be broken down into the different categories described below.

Pain is the body's natural warning system. It is a message sent from the body to the conscious mind to tell us that something is wrong.

Acute pain

This is immediate pain and is usually the result of a physical trauma, such as a fall or a blow, a sprain or break, or inflammation and infection. It is emergency pain and its purpose is to warn. It tells us quickly and directly that something is wrong and that we should do something about it. Acute pain normally resolves itself as healing occurs, but it can become chronic pain after healing.

Chronic pain

This is long-term pain, unlike acute pain, which is normally temporary and disappears with time and treatment. Chronic pain persists after healing has occurred or when the condition causing the pain persists. The purpose of chronic pain for the body is more difficult to ascertain. It is not a simple indicator that something should be done quickly. It is a pain that just will not go away. It is often inexplicable. Sometimes pain is a result of healing—the healing has been successful but in a way that continues to cause pain.

Chronic pain is constant and nagging, and remains in spite of everything you do to ease it. There are many conditions which produce chronic pain including arthritis and rheumatic disorders or long-term diseases such as lupus. Severe chronic pain can be extremely distressing.

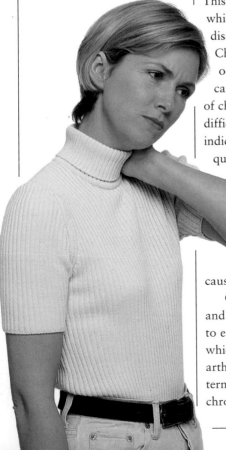

Referred pain

One of the most important features of pain is that it may be "referred." Referred pain is felt some distance from where the pain actually originates. In other words, the site of the pain is not necessarily the source. Osteoarthritis of the hip, for example, causes pain to be experienced in the knee.

Clearly, it is important to discover what is causing the pain in order to be able to treat it effectively and that means being able to identify the real source. But, when the source is not the place where the pain is being felt, this identification can become difficult. This key phenomenon is not clearly understood by nonspecialists and is the main reason for mistakes in the proper and effective relief of pain by people treating themselves. Sometimes such mistakes can be fatal. For example, in very rare cases, pain in the right shoulder can be a symptom of abdominal cancer.

It is vital to seek professional, usually medical, advice for pain that persists, or pain that has no obvious cause.

Emotional pain

Pain is usually thought of as physical. But there is another sort of pain that is equally real. This is emotional "pain" or mental distress—the pain and anguish we feel through our mind and emotions. It is the sort of pain we may experience from being rejected, from bereavement, from problems with relationships, or from the loss of love. External causes, such as the loss of a job or financial worries, can also lead to emotional distress.

One acute form of emotional, or psychological, distress is depression, an all-encompassing term that covers anything from feeling down and sad to extreme mental and emotional agony. Mental pain has its own pain subset that can include nightmares, fears, phobias, and—in the extreme—obsessions and addictions to food, drink, drugs, or sex, for example.

It is important also to recognize that long-term emotional pain can lead to physical symptoms, such as an irritable bowel or migraines. This psychosomatic illness is thus a form of referred pain and can also be difficult to diagnose.

Our response to pain

Physical pain and psychological pain are closely linked. Physical pain can cause psychological effects, ranging from temporary worry to depression, and emotional or mental pain can bring on physical symptoms. It is becoming more widely accepted that the mind and body cannot be treated as separate entities but should be considered as a whole.

This is not only the case with the causes of pain but in the treatment process. Many traditional systems of healing, such as Traditional Chinese medicine, naturopathy, and homeopathy, as well as many conventional doctors specializing in pain management, recognize this link between mind and body. The science of psychoneuroimmunology (PNI) investigates how the mind can help the body to heal, and equally, how the body can affect the mind. The power of the mind can trigger the release of chemicals in the brain, which govern the body's physical state, and these can either act in a positive or negative way.

Equally, addressing aspects of a person's physical state, such as diet and exercise, or even their living or working conditions, can help to ameliorate symptoms of mental or emotional pain.

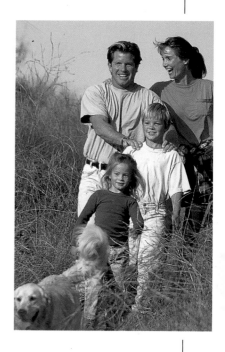

Our tolerance for pain depends on mental attitude, the response of those around us, our ability to control our reactions to pain, and the situation causing the pain.

TYPES OF PAIN

PHYSICAL PAIN		EMOTIONAL PAIN	
ACUTE PAIN	Pain that is of sudden onset and often severe. It may result from an injury or an infection and resolves with recovery and healing.	MENTAL DISTRESS	Can have a clear "external" cause such as any event that would obviously be a source of worry, a deeper emotional loss, or rejection. Some sufferers may only experience a temporary sense of sadness while others may become severely depressed and feel totally incapacitated. Psychological pain is commonly accompanied by physical pain.
CHRONIC PAIN	Pain that continues for a long time and that may have no obvious cause.		
REFERRED PAIN	Pain experienced in a different part of the body from its cause.		

How and why we feel pain

T*he experience of pain and how the body deals with it have only recently begun to be understood in any detail. Researchers around the world have added pieces to the broader picture of an extremely complex and interreactive system. But there are still many problems to be solved.*

Reflex actions protect you by short-circuiting your conscious mind. Your hand will have moved away from a hot surface before you have had time to think about it.

The sensation of physical pain is mediated by a mechanism that works in a way that is similar to other boldily sensations. A stimulus is "felt" in some peripheral part of the body —a pain, such as stubbing your toe, a toothache, or a sensation like touch or smell. This message is conveyed along a nerve to the spinal cord, travels up the spinal cord to the brain, and ends in the specific part of the brain concerned with that particular sensation. This part of the brain interprets the message and it is only here that it is perceived as pain or odor, or heat or cold. If the nerve ending near to the source of the pain is not working, then the pain will not be felt. This is why people whose nerves have degenerated from some cause can undergo considerable damage without noticing.

In leprosy, the protective sheathing of the nerves (the myelin sheath) is damaged by bacteria so that the sufferers may not realize that they have badly hurt a finger, for example.

On the other hand, some neural damage can result in intensified pain. The herpes simplex virus also appears to damage the myelin sheathing of the nerve but, in this case, the lack of insulation can cause one "current" to flow into other adjacent neurons and send more pain sensations to the brain.

The neurons are of many different types and have different functions. They can be wide or narrow and have protective sheaths or not. They also have a wide variety of nerve endings and it appears to be the nerve endings that are specific to different sensations. Pain nerve endings are called nociceptors but, even here, there are different types that are receptive to heat and cold, a mechanical stimulation such as a pinprick, or a more prolonged dull stimulus.

These receptors are excited at the nerve ending either by an electrical action (a change in potential difference caused by movement of charged particles) or a chemical action. Chemicals appear to act by changing the configuration of the cell wall and many different substances can act in this way, some to cause pain and others to dull it.

Intensity of pain

In some cases, an intense pain is what the body needs to protect itself. If we touch a very hot surface, the nerves act extremely quickly to produce a reflex withdrawal of the hand.

But, in other cases, where the body needs its "fight or flight" reactions, it can block out or postpone pain until the emergency is over. Epinephrine is produced to prepare the body for the emergency and appears to be able to inhibit the transmission of pain.

The body can also produce a variety of chemical messengers in response to painful stimuli. Many of these messengers are peptides, which are molecules made up of strings of amino acids. Some will increase the blood flow to the affected area or release histamine, thus initiating repair mechanisms.

Other peptides have been called endorphins or encephalins and these act to inhibit the transmission of pain in the brain by blocking receptors. Over fifty of these peptide messengers have been identified and one puzzle remaining to be solved is why the body needs so many. These substances act in a similar way to opiates without appearing to be addictive and are brought into play in cases of prolonged pain.

Pain gates

One piece of research appears to indicate that a nerve pathway can only support so much activity and that activity in one set of neurons will lower the activity in others. Thus, if some normal sensation is traveling to the brain, it may block out or reduce the activity of the nociceptors.

The pain gate theory provides a tremendous challenge to the usual treatment of pain. Medical treatment for pain, especially for severe chronic pain was, and largely still is, with strong drugs with powerful and sometimes dangerous side effects. The gate theory, however, may make it possible to treat pain in a much gentler way. In particular, it has opened the way for the so-called complementary therapies, which form a large portion of the treatments described in this book.

Attitudes to pain

It is important to think about pain in the right way. It is a natural reaction to fight pain or be angry because one is in pain. But pain should not be suppressed or treated as an enemy. This can lead to extra tensions and unhelpful messages being sent to the body from the mind. Instead, we should learn to listen carefully to the messages which our bodies send us.

By taking advantage of what your doctor can offer, making use of the natural therapies described in this book, and using pacing techniques which avoid the need to break the "pain barrier," you can feel in control of your pain. Accepting pain and working with and through it is not only possible but can be strengthening and even life-enhancing.

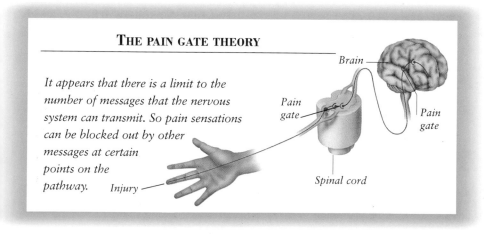

THE PAIN GATE THEORY

It appears that there is a limit to the number of messages that the nervous system can transmit. So pain sensations can be blocked out by other messages at certain points on the pathway.

Brain

Pain gate

Pain gate

Spinal cord

Injury

The nervous system and pain

Pain can be felt in most parts of the body, although some parts have fewer nerve endings than others. The nervous system transmits the sensation of pain from the body to the brain.

The nervous system is made up of a network of complex fibers known as nerves that thread throughout the human body like household wiring. The nerves conduct electrical signals back and forth between the brain and the different parts of the body.

The skin is the organ mostly richly supplied with nerves. It needs to be very sensitive since it is in direct contact with our surroundings. The nervous system transmits the messages it receives from the skin to the brain, where they are interpreted as pain or another form of stimulus. Other parts of the body, such as the muscles, joints, and internal organs, also produce pain signals if they are damaged or overstretched.

The nervous system consists of three different systems that connect to a particular part of the brain:
• the motor nervous system, which controls the muscles of the body
• the sensory nervous system, which channels information from the five main bodily senses of sight, sound, touch, taste, and smell, and the sensation of pain, to your brain
• the autonomic nervous system, which controls automatic functions such as breathing, heartbeat, and digestion.

The most important part of the brain for the central nervous system is the thin outer layer or "grey matter," known as the cerebral cortex. Within the cerebral cortex, the area that controls voluntary muscle

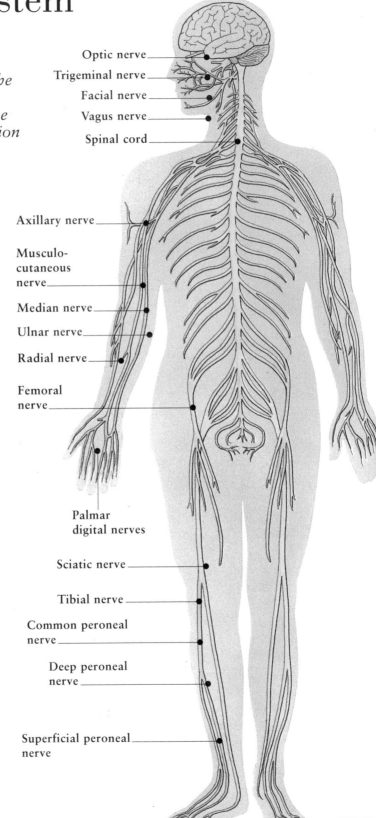

Optic nerve

Trigeminal nerve

Facial nerve

Vagus nerve

Spinal cord

Axillary nerve

Musculo-cutaneous nerve

Median nerve

Ulnar nerve

Radial nerve

Femoral nerve

Palmar digital nerves

Sciatic nerve

Tibial nerve

Common peroneal nerve

Deep peroneal nerve

Superficial peroneal nerve

movement of the limbs is known as the motor area, while the area that receives sensations of pain and touch is the sensory area.

But all except the most simple of signals are relayed to different areas of the brain and can be modified by other messages of inhibition or stimulation.

Nerve pathways

Messages to the brain are carried in nerves or neurons, which run from the periphery of the body into the spinal cord where they are protected by the bones of the spine, called the vertebrae. The spinal cord runs up through the vertebrae to the brain. Signals from the brain are relayed via nerves down the spinal cord to every part of the body and back again.

The brain is protected by the bones of the cranium. Damage to the cranium or vertebrae puts the nervous system at risk and intense pain can be caused by trapping nerves between vertebrae. Sciatica is caused by the trapping of the sciatic nerve at the base of the spine but it is felt as a shooting pain down the leg. It is, therefore, an example of referred pain. Carpal tunnel syndrome or Repetitive Strain Injury is similarly caused by the median nerve, which runs to the fingertips, being trapped by the radial bones of the wrist.

The spinal nerve bundles include nerves of both the motor and sensory systems. If the sensory nerves in the hand pick up a sensation of heat and pain from touching a boiling hot pan, the sensation is relayed via the spinal nerves to the sensory area of the brain. The sensory area sends a signal to the motor area, which transmits a signal back via the spinal cord. This tells the muscles of the hand to let go of the pan quickly.

To pass from cell to cell the messages need to cross gaps known as synapses via the release of chemicals, which pass the impulse across the gap. It is at the synapse that the messages can be modified or controlled.

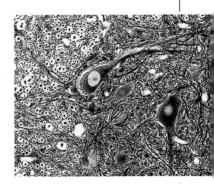

Nerve cells or axons are encased and protected by an outer layer called the myelin sheath, made from a mixture of protein and fats. It acts as an insulator, allowing signals to be transmitted through the axons more rapidly.

AUTONOMIC NERVOUS SYSTEM

The autonomic nervous system controls the body's automatic functions—those that are not normally subject to conscious control, such as breathing and digestion. It is concerned with the maintainance of the normal state of the body and is governed by the cerebral and the hypothalamus (a lobe in the center) areas of the brain. The system comprises the sympathetic nervous system and the parasympathetic nervous system.

The sympathetic system is the "all-action" emergency nervous system, the one that controls the "fight or flight" response programmed into our instincts early in our evolution. Stimulation of the nerves in this system—from fear, anger, or hunger, for example—speeds up the heart and breathing rates, increases the blood supply to the muscles, dilates the pupils of the eye, and reduces digestion and the production of urine and saliva. In contrast, the parasympathetic system is the "rest and recuperation" system. This is the one that takes over during rest or sleep, slowing down the heart and breathing rates and increasing digestion.

The musculoskeletal system and pain

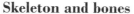

*A*ll the muscles and bones of the body make up the musculo-skeletal system. It gives you your shape, supports you, and allows you to perform mechanical tasks, such as walking, talking, holding, and sitting. It is susceptible to overuse, injury, and inflammation and is therefore a common source of pain.

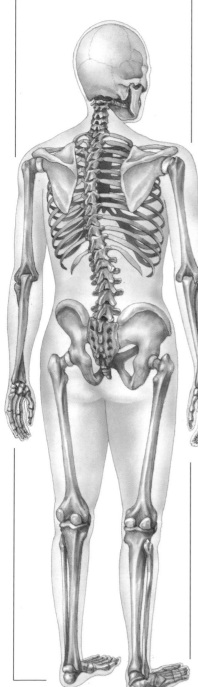

The bones of the skeleton support and protect the body's soft tissues and organs.

Skeleton and bones

The human skeleton is composed of a total of 206 bones divided into two main groups, the axial skeleton and the appendicular skeleton. The axial is the "upright" skeleton—that is, the bones of the chest or thorax, which consist of the spine and the sternum and rib cage. The appendicular skeleton is comprised of all the bones attached to the axial skeleton, mainly the arms and legs but also the skull, which is itself made up of eight different bones.

Bones are the hardest material in the body and are made up of layers of varying density, with the hardest on the outside. Mineral salts, mainly calcium and magnesium, make up approximately two-thirds of bone weight. Some bones, for example, the ribs, breastbone and skull, not only protect vital internal organs but also contain bone marrow where red and white blood cells are chiefly made.

Muscle

Muscular tissue is of three different kinds —skeletal muscle, which attaches to the bones of the skeleton and makes it move, smooth muscle, which is found in the circulatory and digestive systems and is controlled by the autonomic nervous system, and the heart, or cardiac, muscle.

There are 650 skeletal muscles in the human body and they work mainly in pairs, moving bones by alternately contracting and lengthening. For example, when you raise and lower your arm, the muscles of the upper arm (the biceps and triceps) contract and expand to perform the movement. Skeletal muscles, along with the tendons that connect them to the bones, are susceptible to being strained from overuse, cramps, and inflammations.

Smooth muscle makes up the wall of the stomach and gut and is susceptible to hernias when poor muscle tone is caught unawares by a sudden action.

Cardiac muscle is obviously vitally important and has several special characteristics to aid its functioning. Strain on the heart muscle can be felt as chest pain but also as pain in the arms.

Joints and pain

Musculoskeletal pain is rarely caused by bones, unless they are broken or diseased. Pain is usually caused by muscles and their connecting tissues (tendons and ligaments) and, especially, by joints. Hard-working and load-bearing joints, such as those of the neck, back, hips, arms, legs, and feet, are most susceptible, with the knee—the most complex joint in the body—the leading cause of trouble.

Joints are normally classified as synovial, which are free-moving; cartilaginous, which provide limited

TYPES OF SYNOVIAL (FREE-MOVING) JOINTS

JOINT TYPE	MOVEMENT	EXAMPLES OF JOINTS
BALL-AND-SOCKET	All directions	Shoulder, hip
HINGE	One direction only	Elbow, fingers
SADDLE	Two directions	Ankle, thumb
PIVOT	Rotation only	Head to neck
OVOID OR ELLIPSOID	Bending and circular but not rotating	Wrist, finger to hand
CONDYLAR	Mainly one direction but also rotating and locking	Knee
PLANE OR GLIDING	Flat surface movement	Palms, ribs to upper spine

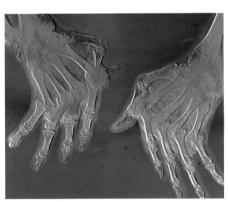

An X ray of inflammation of the synovial membrane around the knuckles caused by rheumatoid arthritis. This makes it painful to straighten the fingers.

In the average male, muscles make up almost half the total body weight, and in women, just over a third of the total body weight. Generally, the larger a muscle is, the more powerful it is.

movement; and fibrous, which have no movement. The area between synovial joints is cushioned by cartilage, which covers the ends of the bones and provides a smooth surface that acts as a shock absorber. The cartilage is contained in a capsule lined by the synovial membrane. This produces a lubricant known as synovial fluid. Inflammation of the synovial membrane is the most frequent cause of joint pain, and may lead to damage of all the vital component parts of joints. This is what happens, for example, in cases of rheumatoid or systemic arthritis.

Digestive and urinary systems and pain

These two independent but connected systems are responsible for converting food and liquid into energy and expelling waste. The organs work hard and continuously during the life of a living being and are often abused and overloaded.

The digestive and urinary systems consist of a series of about a dozen organs from the mouth to the groin. These organs are subject to abuse when people do not regulate their intake of food and drink. They are not well supplied with nerve endings and pain in these organs can be difficult to identify and treat.

The digestive system

From the mouth to the gut, food and drink follow the pathway described in the diagram opposite and are broken down and digested in a series of processes by different organs. These organs are also responsible for the excretion of the body's waste materials, such as worn-out tissue cells, and of toxins, that is, materials which the body cannot use.

The digestive system is resilient and hard-working. Nevertheless, much commonly experienced pain and disease occurs in this tract. This broadly stems from two causes: first, the digestive process itself needs energy to operate and too often our lifestyles prevent us from giving it time to function smoothly. Indigestion and irritable bowel syndrome often stem from this, coupled with stress. Secondly, people suffer from eating disorders, such as anorexia or bulimia, or simply eat or drink toxins like alcohol or caffeine that actually damage the organs.

One malfunction of the digestive organs that can cause acute pain is the formation of stones. Several organs, including the gallbladder and kidney, will produce stones if the balance of material passing through them is upset. Gallstones are formed by a crystallization of cholesterol if the liver and gallbladder cannot deal with an excess fat intake.

The appendix appears to be a vestigial organ that human beings no longer need. Stray food matter or bacteria can become lodged there and cause appendicitis. This can be difficult to diagnose; the pain may occur in the upper or lower abdomen and can be mistaken for other digestive or urinary tract disorders.

The urinary system

The urinary system consists of the kidneys, ureter, bladder, and urethra. The kidneys filter the blood and remove toxins, while also maintaining the body's balance of water, salts, and hormones. Damage to the kidneys is extremely serious and is sometimes irreparable.

From the kidneys, urine passes down the ureter into the bladder and from there is expelled via another thin tube known as the urethra. The lower urinary tract is susceptible to infections, such as cystitis, when bacteria, often from the gut, enter via the urethra and can cause painful and irritable inflammations, especially in women.

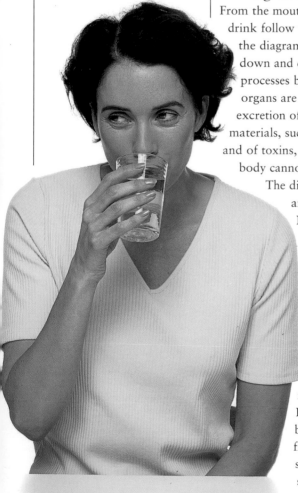

Drinking plenty of water helps to clear waste materials from the body and replaces lost moisture.

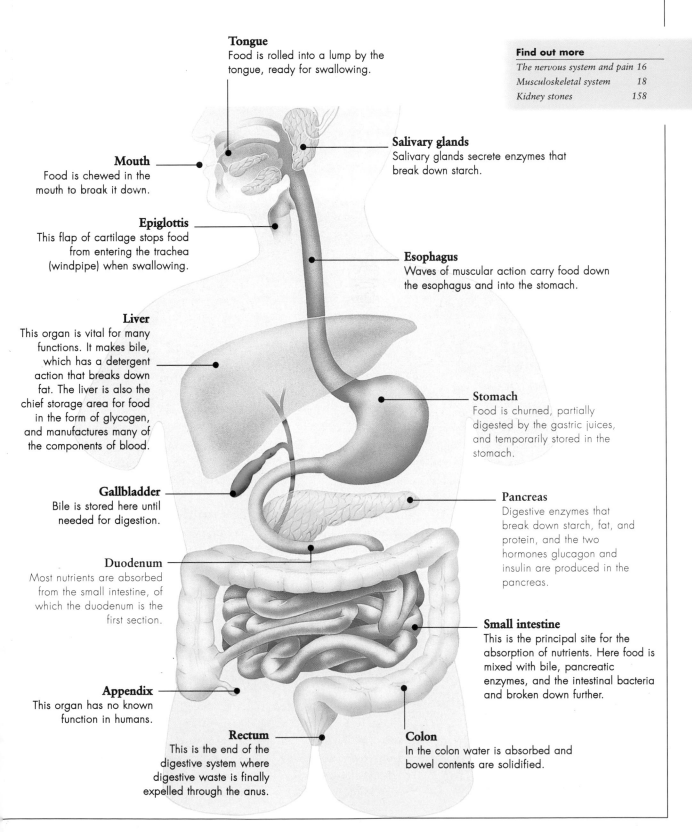

Tongue
Food is rolled into a lump by the tongue, ready for swallowing.

Mouth
Food is chewed in the mouth to break it down.

Salivary glands
Salivary glands secrete enzymes that break down starch.

Epiglottis
This flap of cartilage stops food from entering the trachea (windpipe) when swallowing.

Esophagus
Waves of muscular action carry food down the esophagus and into the stomach.

Liver
This organ is vital for many functions. It makes bile, which has a detergent action that breaks down fat. The liver is also the chief storage area for food in the form of glycogen, and manufactures many of the components of blood.

Stomach
Food is churned, partially digested by the gastric juices, and temporarily stored in the stomach.

Gallbladder
Bile is stored here until needed for digestion.

Pancreas
Digestive enzymes that break down starch, fat, and protein, and the two hormones glucagon and insulin are produced in the pancreas.

Duodenum
Most nutrients are absorbed from the small intestine, of which the duodenum is the first section.

Small intestine
This is the principal site for the absorption of nutrients. Here food is mixed with bile, pancreatic enzymes, and the intestinal bacteria and broken down further.

Appendix
This organ has no known function in humans.

Rectum
This is the end of the digestive system where digestive waste is finally expelled through the anus.

Colon
In the colon water is absorbed and bowel contents are solidified.

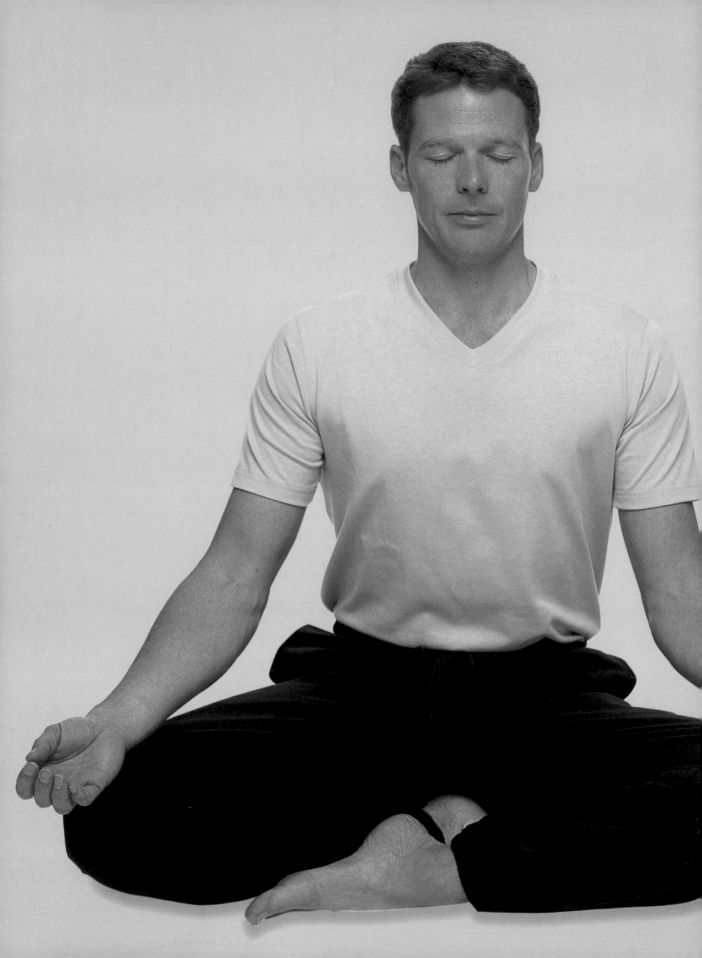

2

APPROACHES TO

PAIN RELIEF

Pain varies from that produced by an acute malfunction to nagging minor irritation. As a result, different approaches to pain relief are appropriate for different conditions. Conventional medicine has tended to rely on the prescription of powerful drugs to alleviate symptoms; they may not address the cause of the problem and may be too harsh for the body.

Complementary therapies provide an approach in which the sufferer can take charge of his or her own well-being. An accurate medical diagnosis of the cause of pain is always advisable and, for serious illness, complementary therapies should be practiced alongside conventional treatment.

Complementary medicine

A lternative therapies provide treatments that are not found within conventional medicine, but can be used alongside conventional treatments. They include Traditional Chinese Medicine, naturopathy, shamanic medicine, traditional European folk and herbal medicine, and also various forms of modern "New Age" medicine.

Aromatherapy oils can be used, usually diluted in a base oil, for a soothing massage, a relaxing bath, in a burner to scent a room, or breathed in as an infusion to clear your lungs and nasal passages.

Nonconventional medicine is not a defined area but an ever-widening collection of therapies. In recent years the description "complementary" has come to mean that many of the therapies and treatments are not a replacement for conventional medicine but are complementary to it; that is, they work in partnership with conventional medicine, rather than instead of it.

Some therapists claim that they are offering an alternative to conventional medicine but most now accept the term complementary medicine to describe their methods of treatment.

"Traditional medicine" in this context is a term used to describe the areas of traditional folk or native medicine from various cultures. Such medicine usually has a history of several hundred years but this in itself should not be taken as proof of its efficacy.

Users should approach all forms of medical treatment with a critical eye. Conventional Western medicine has developed over the last 150 years as techniques of isolating drugs and of performing more accurate surgery have grown out of herbalism and older surgical practices.

The holistic approach

The fundamental philosophy of complementary medicine is, or should be, exactly what is at the core of good conventional medicine: To use the gentlest approach; to avoid dangerous and traumatic procedures; and to treat the patient holistically. Patients are viewed as "whole" individuals, composed of body, mind, and emotions, who may be creating their own illness for some reason but who can also take an active part in their own well-being and recovery after illness.

General principles

Although complementary medicine is a collection of widely different treatments, most complementary therapists understand, accept, and operate under the following principles:

• A human being is a subtle and complex blend of body, mind, and emotions. A problem in any of these areas may cause or contribute to health problems. Each individual is a fully integrated "whole," not a random collection of moving parts.

• Good health is a state of emotional, mental, spiritual, and physical balance. Balance is fundamental to the notion of health, and ill-health is the result of imbalance or "disease."

• Environmental and social factors have a bearing on a person's physical and emotional makeup and therefore can impact on their health.

• Treating the root causes of a problem is

more important than treating the immediate symptoms. Treating only the symptoms may mask the underlying problem, so that it reappears later as something more serious.

• Each person is an individual and cannot be treated in exactly the same way as another person. A complementary therapist will generally want to know more about you than a conventional medical practitioner.

• The body has a natural ability to heal itself and return to stability but healing is quicker and more effective if the person takes responsibility for his or her own health and takes an active part in the healing process.

Effectiveness of complementary therapies

People often turn to a complementary therapist as a last resort, having tried the conventional route and found it unsatisfactory, but it is better in many cases to include complementary medicine as an integral part of your treatment regime. Those people who do often experience a higher level of satisfaction. This can derive both from an actual amelioration of their condition and from the experience of a better quality of care than they experience from the normal medical treatment. Patients have found that treatments, such as osteopathy, chiropractic, acupuncture, herbalism, homeopathy, massage, aromatherapy, reflexology, and healing are effective in treating pain.

In recent years there has been a rapid rise in the numbers of doctors and nurses using or recommending complementary therapies for pain. However, many practitioners of conventional medicine continue to be wary of complementary

therapies. This is because most often it cannot be shown why a treatment has worked and the lack of controlled, experimental proof is alien to the scientific approach. Secondly, if one treatment does not work, patients may try something different and this too contradicts conventional medicine's scheme of specific treatments for specific complaints.

The recent popularity of nonconventional medicine has resulted in a host of new treatments entering the "menu" of pain therapies. These range from well-known approaches, such as acupuncture, osteopathy, and homeopathy, to lesser-known, recently introduced, and unvalidated therapies. Some of these are unlikely to stand the test of time.

It is also true that many practitioners have no formal training or qualifications. They may still offer effective treatment but patients should bear this in mind when seeking out a practitioner. Many of the older treatments now have training courses and professional bodies regulating their practice. All the therapies discussed in this book have been proven to be successful in treating pain.

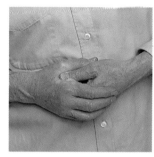

Acupressure is a popular self-help therapy. It is based on the same principles as acupuncture but relies on pressure applied to points on the skin rather than the insertion of needles.

THE NATURAL HEALING FORCE

Many people believe that there is a natural healing force or energy in the universe. The Chinese call it qi *or* chi *(pronounced "chee"), the Japanese call it* ki, *and Indians call it* prana. *In the West it used to be called by its Latin description* vis medicatrix naturae, *meaning "natural healing force," but this has been simplified to the more usual "life force" today. Most complementary therapists believe that anyone can make use of this force and that a skilled practitioner can activate it in the patient or help the patient to activate it in themselves.*

Types of complementary therapy

Complementary therapies fall roughly into two main categories: physical therapies and psychological therapies. Some practitioners believe there is a third category, which they refer to as energy therapies.

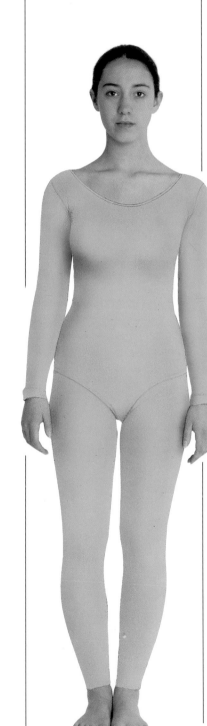

A therapy may work through physical manipulation or activity or by introducing the patient to alternative medicines, such as herbal or homeopathic substances, or by treating the patient's mental state through visualization, through music, or meditation. Many patients find that they like to use more than one therapy and approach their problem in different ways. But most complementary practitioners will look at all aspects of their patients.

Physical therapies

These therapies approach the patient primarily through the body. The treatment can either be passive on the part of the patient, such as in massage or reflexology, or active, as in yoga or t'ai chi. Some, like yoga, also emphasize the patient's mental state, while physiotherapy, for example, is more purely physical.

Physical therapies also include those that offer the patient nontraditional medicines, such as herbal medicines. Dietary therapies also concentrate on achieving the right balance of food intake. Aromatherapy, which uses natural fragrant oils to induce mental states, is also partly a physical therapy, in that the patient is absorbing the fragrances through their senses and that this may be via massage.

Yoga works by treating the mind and body together in physical exercises that, among other things, improve posture.

Psychological therapies

Psychological therapies address mental and emotional states. For patients who are suffering physical pain as well as those whose illness arises from stress or emotional pain, psychological therapies are used to produce relaxation, both physical and mental.

Again, these treatments can be active or passive. Patients can listen to or make music, paint, or be guided through meditation or visualization techniques.

Mental and emotional states of a more serious nature are treated with therapies, such as counseling, psychotherapy, and hypnotherapy for severe emotional distress, obsessions, phobias, and addictions.

Energy therapies

The body's subtle or hidden "energy field" or "life force" is addressed through energy therapies. The energy is said to be channeled in pathways, called meridians in Chinese medicine, and in yoga there are energy centers, called chakras, which are used to focus different sorts of energy.

Energy therapies are often based on Eastern ideas of health and disease (or dis-ease) and work on the basis that illness is the result of an imbalance or interruption in the body's natural energy or "life force" at a very fine or subtle level. Oriental ideas of "energy" are increasingly being used in the treatment of pain. These therapies include acupuncture, acupressure, and "faith healing."

COMPLEMENTARY THERAPIES HELPFUL FOR PAIN

PHYSICAL THERAPIES	Alexander technique
	Aromatherapy
	Electromagnetic therapy
	Herbalism
	Manipulation (including
	   chiropractic, cranial
	   osteopathy, and
	   osteopathy)
		Massage
		Naturopathy (including
		   hydrotherapy)
		Nutritional and dietary
		   therapy
		Reflexology
		T'ai chi
		Yoga

PSYCHOLOGICAL THERAPIES	Biofeedback Counseling Hypnotherapy	Meditation Psychotherapy Relaxation and visualization
ENERGY THERAPIES	Acupuncture Homeopathy	Reflexology Shiatsu

How complementary medicine is practiced

Complementary medical techniques vary in the depth of knowledge needed to try them. For some therapies, the patient needs expert practitioner treatment. Within this category are the manipulation therapies, such as osteopathy, Rolfing, and chiropractic, and the psychological therapies, such as counseling, hypnotherapy, and psychotherapy.

Some therapies fall into an "in between" category, in that, initially, they require expert diagnosis and treatment or require that the patient receive training before they can carry out the therapy correctly at home. This category includes movement therapies like the Alexander technique, as well as therapies such as Chinese herbalism.

In the third category are those that you can safely do at home without expert supervision, such as physical therapies like aromatherapy, some dietary therapies, movement therapies, like yoga and t'ai chi, energy therapies, such as shiatsu, and psychological therapies like meditation.

All self-administered therapy should be approached with common sense and moderation.

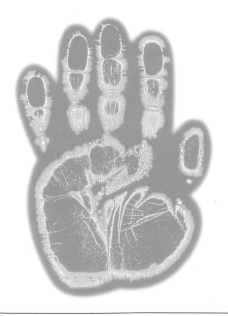

Kirlian photography registers the response of the body to an electric signal. It is an energy-based diagnostic therapy that claims to measure and analyze the energy fields in the body. The glowing outline around the hand is known as the aura.

What to expect from a therapist

M ost natural health practitioners will give you a lot more time than you may be used to getting from your family doctor. A first visit can last from half an hour to two hours, enabling the therapist to learn as much about you and your life as he or she needs in order to suggest the best possible treatment.

A complementary therapist will pay considerable attention to the way you are feeling at the time of your appointment, and you will probably be treated for that before the therapist attempts to treat other symptoms. For example, if you arrive for your appointment with cold or flu symptoms, you will probably be treated for them, rather than for the pain. This is because therapists believe that there is a reason for the infection and it must be cleared first. Therapists also believe that such conditions may also be linked in some way to the problem causing the pain.

Taking responsibility for your own health may include finding out more about the complaint you are suffering from or the treatment you are receiving.

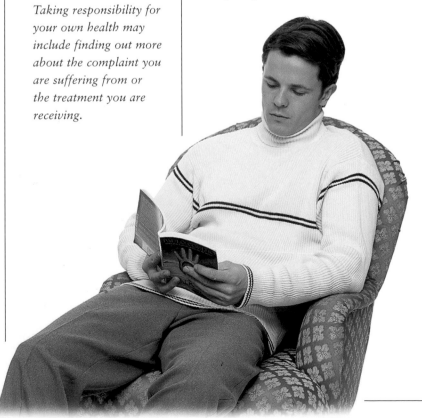

You are likely to find this a common approach, whether you are seeing an osteopath for backache, a reflexologist for an irritable bowel, an aromatherapist for stress, or an acupuncturist for migraines. Complementary therapists will adapt the treatment to suit the circumstances of each individual visit in the belief that by doing so they are encouraging the body to heal itself in the best way possible.

Taking responsibility

Most complementary therapists believe that someone who has sought them out wants to take responsibility for his or her own health and to participate in the process of getting well, instead of just being a passive recipient of treatment. This approach is very different from the conventional medical principle of treating physical symptoms in isolation, although orthodox doctors are increasingly taking psychological factors into account in such areas as pain management, rehabilitation after a heart attack, or chronic fatigue.

Truly holistic therapists treat the individual as a complex mixture of interacting influences, rather than just representative of a textbook problem requiring a textbook solution.

Actively participating in your own healing and restoring your own health has been shown to be an important factor in the success of most complementary therapies. For this reason a good practitioner will always encourage you to do this.

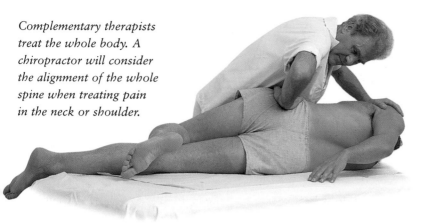

Complementary therapists treat the whole body. A chiropractor will consider the alignment of the whole spine when treating pain in the neck or shoulder.

TAKING A CASE HISTORY

Before treatment, the first concern of any good therapist is to find out what is wrong with you and, more importantly, why you are ill. To do this, a therapist will go through a process known as history taking. Its basic purpose is to discover as much about you as possible. This will include your personality and temperament as well as your physical state.

The full history taking will occur on your first visit to a therapist and will take from approximately half an hour to an hour. During this time you should be prepared for questions and investigative methods that go far beyond what your conventional medical practitioner requires.

Your particular condition may be the result of psychological problems as much as, or possibly even more than, any physical problems. For this reason you will be asked questions about your mental and emotional state as well as your physical ailment. This holistic diagnosis is usually achieved by a long and thorough question-and-answer session during which the therapist will ask you not only about the precise symptoms of your complaint but also about your lifestyle, diet, social circumstances, relationships, bowel habits, sleep patterns, and so on. Skilled therapists will also note your body language as you respond to questions—how you sit, what you do with your hands, where you look—because this may reveal more about you than what you say or do not say.

Practitioners in some disciplines, such as Traditional Chinese Medicine and Ayurvedic medicine will also examine your tongue, feel your pulses (unlike in orthodox medicine, there are several), and examine your urine and stools. Others, particularly in Western countries, may use techniques, such as examining the irises of the eyes (iridology), dowsing with a pendulum, and using Kirlian or aura diagnosis, or hair analysis.

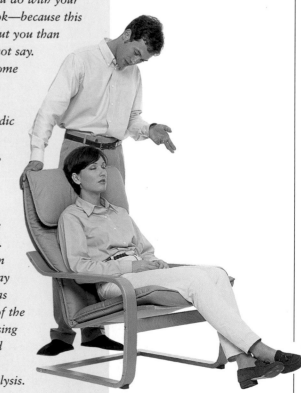

Dietary therapy

The aim of dietary therapy is to maximize health through nutrition. A dietary therapist will analyze the existing diet and then draw up a plan of what the client should be eating to improve their overall health. Foods that may have had a detrimental effect on the client's health will be cut out.

Fresh fruits and vegetables contain large amounts of vitamins and minerals. Drinking fresh fruit juice is a good way of taking in these essential nutrients.

There are many diets, based on various principles, that have been designed to promote health and that claim to be effective in alleviating some painful conditions. They include the mono diet, the Hay diet, the Gerson diet, and the macrobiotic diet. Specific dietary recommendations have also been matched to specific illnesses, such as asthma, migraine, and arthritis. Sufferers from these and others illnesses should monitor their pain history and diet carefully and may be able to discover for themselves a helpful regime. Any diet should be examined carefully to see that it includes all necessary nutrients and should be followed with caution.

Macrobiotic diet

The macrobiotic or "yin-yang" diet aims to return the body to its ideal yin-yang energy balance with foods containing yin and yang energies.

Yang is the active hot side of our nature; yin is the cool, peaceful aspect. Yang foods include cereal grains, root vegetables, and legumes, while yin foods include leafy vegetables, nuts and seeds, and fruit.

Macrobiotics also emphasizes that foods should be organically and locally produced and eaten in their proper seasons.

The mono diet

It is claimed that mono diets, or single-food diets, promote the "cleansing" of the digestive system through the consumption of only one type of fruit or vegetable for two days or more. The food is usually puréed or juiced. Grapes, apples, carrots, beets, and cabbage are commonly used.

Food combining diet (Hay diet)

Devised by Dr. William Hay, an American surgeon, the food combining diet involves not eating starchy foods, such as pasta, bread, and potatoes at the same time as protein foods, such as meat, fish, and dairy foods. The theory is that starch and proteins are "converted" in the digestive tract by different chemical processes and eating them together means that neither is converted properly. The diet has a reputation for effectively treating pain caused by arthritis and digestive problems.

Gerson diet

Pioneered by Dr. Max Gerson, an American doctor, the Gerson diet claims to help prevent cancer. The diet includes organically grown fruit and vegetables, particularly green leafy vegetables, such as cabbage, brussels sprouts, and broccoli, which contain chemicals called indoles.

Indoles deactivate estrogen, which may be implicated in certain types of

DIETARY AND NUTRITIONAL THERAPY

Dietary and nutritional therapies are not the same. Dietary therapy emphasizes correct eating and drinking for health, while nutritional therapy is concerned with the use of nutritional or food supplements to treat existing health problems.

Dietary therapists, or dietitians, advise on what you should or should not eat, while nutritional therapists specialize in the recommendation of specific doses of vitamins and minerals for healing purposes.

Although there is a growing overlap between the two therapies, and it is possible that they may become a single discipline at some point in the future, important differences do exist.

For example, dietitians do not recommend high doses of vitamins and minerals for the purposes of treating illnesses because few dietitians accept the need for extra nutrients if a healthy, balanced diet is followed.

Conversely, nutritionists, even though they support the idea of healthy eating, believe that the average Western diet does not contain all the nutrients the body needs, attributing this largely to modern methods of food production, which make most foods low in nutrients or altogether lacking in nutrients. Nutritionists recommend that these missing nutrients should be provided through the intake of various vitamin, mineral, and other food supplements.

cancer, and this may indicate there is some justification for the Gerson diet.

Fasting

Though not all doctors agree, a fast of no longer than 24 hours, carried out under proper advice and supervision, is an effective way of clearing toxins out of the body.

Diets for specific illnesses

Many chronic illnesses can be alleviated by attention to the diet. This may be different for different patients but it seems that, generally, a low-fat, low-protein diet can ease pain from rheumatoid arthritis. Migraine sufferers should avoid cheese, chocolate, and wine. Asthma patients should try to ascertain which foods they react badly to and avoid foods containing sulfites, such as wine and beer.

HAIR MINERAL ANALYSIS

Some nutritional therapists use samples of hair to detect mineral deficiencies within the body. This technique involves sending a hair sample to a laboratory for analysis. At the laboratory the hair sample is cut into segments, which are analyzed to detect the presence or absence of specific substances. Some laboratories will then suggest various mineral supplement products that should be taken by the client in order to redress the balance and will sell them to the client.

Laboratories generally charge very high prices for analysis and many specialists doubt the value of such testing. Hair mineral content may not be an accurate reflection of the state of the body and different laboratories have been shown to produce conflicting results on the same samples of hair.

Also, hair is affected by the shampoos and other products we use and the processes used by hairdressers and may not be a true indication of our internal state. For this reason, we should not rely on hair analysis alone to determine the mineral content of the body.

Dietary therapy

GUIDE TO HEALTHY EATING AND DRINKING			
FOODS	REGULARLY	SOMETIMES	AVOID
CAKES AND COOKIES		Cakes, desserts, and cookies made with polyunsaturated fats, sorbets and low-fat ice cream	Ready-made cakes and cookies, cream cakes, full-fat ice cream
CEREALS AND BREAD	Whole-wheat flour, oats, whole-wheat pasta, brown rice, sugar- and salt-free cereals	Refined pasta, white rice, white bread, crackers, white flour products	Croissants, brioches, and pastries
DAIRY AND EGG PRODUCTS	Nonfat milk, egg white, low-fat yogurt, low-fat cottage cheese	Low-fat milk, medium- and half-fat cheeses, egg yolks	Yogurt made with whole milk, cream, full-fat cheeses, coffee creamers
DRINKS AND SOUPS	Water, fruit juice, low-fat soups, tea	Alcohol, coffee, malted drinks, and low-fat hot chocolate	Creamy soups, whole-milk drinks
FATS AND OILS	Olive oil	Polyunsaturated oils and margarines, e.g. sunflower oil, corn oil, and low-fat spreads	Butter, lard, ghee
FISH	Sardines, tuna, salmon, mackerel, trout, white fish such as cod or haddock		Fried fish in batter
FRUIT AND VEGETABLES	Fresh or frozen fruits and vegetables; beans, lentils and other legumes	French fries cooked in polyunsaturated oil, avocados	Potato chips, french fries
MEAT	Skinless chicken and turkey	Lean beef, pork, lamb, liver, kidney, or organ meats	Fatty meat, sausages, meat pies, salamis, duck, pâté
DRESSINGS, PRESERVES, AND CANDIES	Herbs, mustard, sugar-free jams	Low-fat salad dressing and mayonnaise, sugar-filled jams, marmalade, dark chocolate	Cream-based dressings and mayonnaise, sugar, milk chocolate, honey, candies

Dietary therapists recommend a diet high in raw fruit, vegetables, and fiber but low in saturated fat, salt, and sugar. This chart shows which foods you should eat regularly, which you can have on occasion, and which to avoid.

Nutritional therapy

W*ith the discovery of vitamin A in 1913, scientists recognized the vital part these compounds play in nutrition. Dietary supplements have become more widespread with the identification of many more essential vitamins.*

Vitamins play an essential part in the body's metabolism. There are about 15 of them, but vitamin B is usually referred to as vitamin B complex because it consists of a group of related compounds. The body is able to synthesize some vitamins from foodstuffs; others must be obtained whole from the diet. The vitamins can be divided into those that are soluble in fat and those that are water-soluble. The fat-soluble ones, A, D, E, and K can be stored in the body, but the water-soluble ones, B and C, cannot be stored and therefore need to be supplied regularly. Furthermore, because they are soluble in water, they are often lost in the cooking process. If vitamins that the body puts into storage are taken in excess, they can be harmful, while generally speaking, the body will simply excrete excess amounts of vitamins B and C.

Nutritional therapy is based on the fact that deficiencies of various nutrients in the body will cause malfunctions, ranging from scurvy (lack of vitamin C) to anemia (which may be lack of iron, or vitamins B, C, or E). The missing vitamins can either be supplied by balancing the diet or by taking vitamin supplements. During illness the body requires more nutrients to allow it to fight against the condition and repair its cells sufficiently.

A nutritional therapist will analyze your diet, your current state of health, and your lifestyle. Armed with this information, he or she will advise dietary changes and therapeutic doses of various nutritional supplements.

Megavitamin therapy

When used for healing, rather than for general health, the supplement doses recommended can sometimes be extremely high. For example, doses of 1,000 mg or more of vitamin C may be recommended to fight disease, although the amount recommended by authorities for normal daily consumption is just 60 mg. Megavitamin therapy is not usually recommended except on the advice of qualified practitioners because it is possible to overdose. However, taking vitamin and mineral supplements in the doses recommended on the labels is safe (see chart overleaf, page 35).

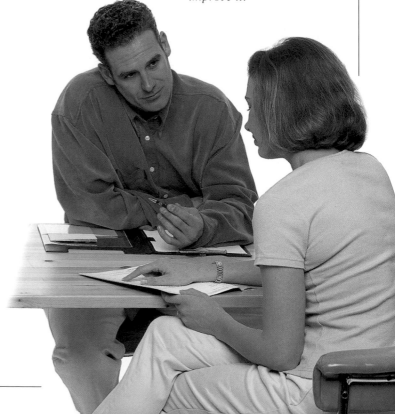

A nutritionist will analyze everything you eat to determine the healthiness —or otherwise—of your diet. He or she will then make recommendations to improve it.

Nutritional therapy

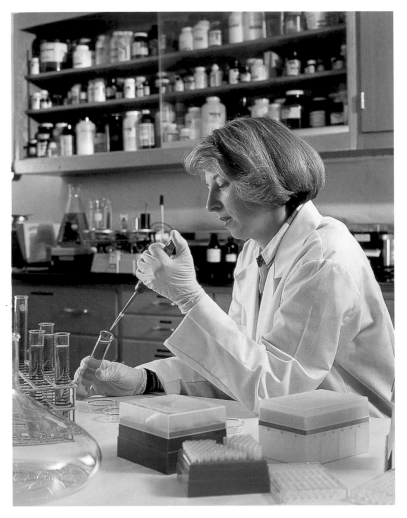

Nutritional deficiencies in the diet can be identified by analysis of body fluids.

usually be taken as a complex because there are more than a dozen of them and they work by complementing each other.

When taking supplements, you should follow these guidelines:

• Take supplements with or just after a meal.

• If taking a number of supplements, divide them equally between meals—for example, half at breakfast and half at lunch, or a third at breakfast, lunch, and dinner—and spread the combination evenly throughout the day. Do not take all the vitamin C in the morning and all the B-complex in the evening since these cannot be stored by the body for later use. If they are surplus to requirements they are eliminated from the body.

• If self-dosing, always follow the guidelines for doses written on the labels. Taking one or more combination supplement with a daily multivitamin and mineral supplement may mean you are overdosing.

• Seek the advice of a trained therapist if you want to take large doses of any supplements. Their effects can vary: for example, B vitamins taken late at night can cause restlessness while multiminerals can aid sleep. Moreover, high doses of some supplements taken over a long time or at the wrong time (such as during pregnancy) can be toxic. Examples are vitamin A, zinc, iron, and selenium.

• Expect to feel benefits within the first three months. See a nutritional therapist if no benefits are experienced.

• Stop taking the supplements and see a therapist if you start to feel unwell or have side effects or unusual symptoms, such as nausea or headaches.

• For a specific condition it is advisable to seek the expert advice of a qualified nutritional therapist.

Generally, supplements should be taken regularly over a period of weeks, months, or even years, although a quick boost of vitamin C can help to give the immune system a boost.

Taking a high quality multivitamin and mineral supplement is the best way of ensuring you get a balance of nutrients. Supplementing with one vitamin or mineral on its own is not as effective as taking several nutrients together. Many nutrients need others to be effective. For example, vitamin C needs zinc to work properly and the B vitamins should

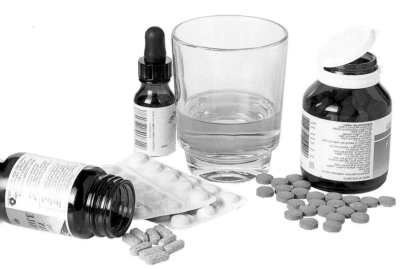

Supplement tablets are dense, compressed concentrations of ingredients. Capsules contain the ingredients in a looser form and tinctures provide them as a liquid.

DAILY REQUIREMENTS FOR VITAMINS AND MINERALS

VITAMIN	RDA (M/W)	RNI (M/W)	MINERAL	RDA (M/W)	RNI (M/W)
A	1000/800 µg	1,000/800 µg	CALCIUM	1,000-1,200 mg	800/700-800 mg
B_1 (thiamin)	1.2/1.1 mg	0.8-1.3/0.8-0.9 mg	IODINE	150 µg	160 µg/160 µg
B_2 (riboflavin)	1.3/1.1 mg	1.3/1.1 mg	IRON	10/15 mg	9-10/13 mg
B_3 (niacin)	16/14 mg	14-23/14-16 mg	MAGNESIUM	420/320 mg	230-250/200-210 mg
B_6	1.3-1.7/1.3-1.5 mg	No RNI	PHOSPHORUS	700 mg	1,000/850 mg
B_{12}	2.4/2.4 µg	1.0/1.0 µg	ZINC	15/12 mg	12/9 mg
C	60/60 mg	40/30 mg	COPPER	No RDA	No RNI
D	5-10/5-10 µg	2.5/2.5 µg	CHROMIUM	No RDA	No RNI
E	10/8 mg	9-10/6-7 mg	MANGANESE	No RDA	No RNI
B_7 (biotin)	No RDA	No RNI	MOLYBDENUM	No RDA	No RNI
B_9 (folic acid)	400/400 µg	220-230/180-200 µg	SELENIUM	No RDA	No RNI
B_5 (pantothenic acid)	No RDA	No RNI			

mg = milligram µg = microgram

M = healthy men W = healthy women.
RDA = Recommended dietary allowance (U.S.).
RNI = Recommended nutrient intakes (Canada).
These requirements vary with age, gender, and physique. People may have different requirements at different times, so seek advice before deciding on a dosage. Since supplements can be taken in excessive amounts, the National Academy of Sciences has produced a list of Tolerable Upper Intake Levels for various nutrients including Calcium – 2,500 mg, Vitamin D – 2,000 I.U. (International Units), Niacin – 35 mg, Vitamin B_6 – 100 mg, and B_9 (folic acid) – 1,000 µg. It is recommended that adults do not exceed these daily limits when taking these vitamins and minerals.

Aromatherapy

Oils distilled from a variety of plants are believed to have healing properties. These concentrated oils are known as essential oils and are each characterized by strong, individual, and pleasant fragrances.

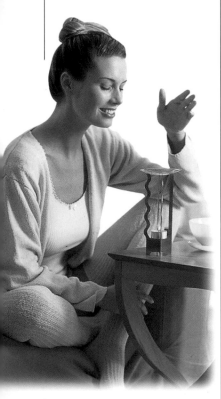

Essential oils can be inhaled into the body from a burner or vaporizer.

The use of essential oils in massages is a practice going back thousands of years. The term aromatherapy was first used in the 1920s by the French chemist René-Maurice Gattefossé who was interested in the healing properties of plants. The oils are usually massaged onto the skin or are inhaled, although a few can be taken internally.

Using essential oils

Aromatherapy oils contain concentrated plant compounds that can cause a severe skin reaction if used without first diluting them with a carrier oil, such as almond, grapeseed, or sunflower oil. They can be safely used if you follow these rules:
• Always follow the directions on the bottle. Usually the dosage is to dilute 25 drops of essential oil to 50 ml of carrier oil, although a more diluted formula will be advised for tender parts of the body, such as the face or genitals. Do not apply to the genital area unless advised to do so by a qualified aromatherapy practitioner.
• Avoid the eye area. Never put oils into the ears unless advised by a practitioner.
• Oils should never be taken internally unless under expert supervision.
• Certain oils are unsuitable for young children and pregnant women (cedarwood, for example) and should not be used without the advice of a fully qualified aromatherapist.
• Never use aromatherapy as a substitute for receiving a proper diagnosis or medical care for an ailment.
• The quality of oils varies widely. Generally, cheaper oils are of poor quality and are likely to be less effective.

THERAPEUTIC USE

Essential oils can act either by inhalation or by penetration via the skin. Experts differ on how much is actually absorbed into the body and claim that an aromatherapy massage is beneficial only as a pleasant relaxant. But therapists believe the effect is more than that, claiming that the aromas can improve emotional and mental well-being by acting directly on the brain via the nose or improve certain conditions of the skin or metabolism. For some people, the oils inhaled from a burner or in the bath can provide a valuble counter to stress and anxiety.

Massages with essential oils can help a wide range of pain problems ranging from angina or arthritis to migraines and backaches. As well as working like a medicinal herb, the oils can also improve muscle tone and promote relaxation, thus helping to ease tension and increase mobility. The soothing effect of an aromatherapy massage can also help ease depression, emotional stress, and fatigue.

Find out more

Massage	56
Reflexology	74

ESSENTIAL OILS AND THEIR THERAPEUTIC USES

ACTION	OIL	CONDITIONS
CALMING	Sandalwood	Sore skin, lack of sexual desire
	Myrrh	Nerve pain (neuralgia, neuritis), chilblains, frostbite
	Neroli	Backache, PMS, headache, poor circulation, insomnia, depression
	Jasmine	Depression, childbirth, lack of sexual desire
	Rose	Sore throat, sinusitis, poor circulation, PMS, depression, insomnia
BALANCING	Lavender	Headache, insomnia, depression, bruises and swelling, insect bites
	Geranium	Skin pain (cuts, sores, bruises, athlete's foot, insect bites)
	Chamomile	Heartburn, PMS, hay fever, skin conditions, muscle and nerve pain
	Cypress	Muscle, joint and tendon pain
	Rosemary	Joint pain, breathing problems, physical/mental fatigue
	Marjoram	Headache, sore throat, PMS, poor circulation, yeast infections, insomnia
STIMULATING	Eucalyptus	Sinusitis, muscle, joint, and tendon pain
	Hyssop	Sinusitis, coughs, eczema, dermatitis
	Juniper	Eczema, cystitis, prostatitis, urethritis, kidney stones
	Pine	Sinusitis, chest pain from breathing problems, hyperventilation
	Tea tree	Sore throat, menstrual pain, vaginitis, pelvic infection; can also be applied as an antiseptic

The above list outlines the most popular and effective oils for a variety of aches and pains. These oils are easy to find and safe to use for the conditions described, provided they are not used as a substitute for medical treatment.

Acupressure and pressure techniques

A cupressure is a simple form of pain control that uses finger or hand pressure on the acupuncture points of the body. It can be practiced at home to relieve pain once the pressure points and techniques have been learned.

Acupressure is often referred to as acupuncture without needles because it uses the acupuncture points of the body. It is a method of healing which we have learned from the East. Practitioners there believe that the pressure points lie along meridians, or energy flowlines in the body. The meridians are named after the organ thought to be affected by the pressure points along it.

Pain caused by problems of the musculoskeletal system, especially tension, is said to respond particularly well to acupressure. Self-help acupressure is most effective as a first-aid technique for acute pain, such as that caused by migraines or fibrositis, and for nausea attacks due to motion sickness. For chronic conditions, treatment by a trained therapist is necessary.

OTHER PRESSURE TECHNIQUES

Most forms of acupressure in use today were developed in Japan. The best known variation is shiatsu but other forms are used, each with their own techniques. They are usually carried out by a trained therapist.

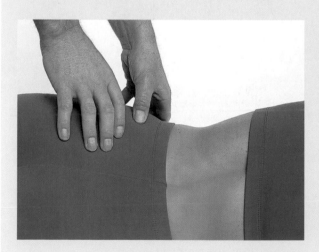

SHIATSU: *The particular characteristic of shiatsu is the rhythmic use of pressure for a few seconds up to a few minutes on special points or "tsubos" located along the energy channels or meridians. Practitioners also use physiotherapy techniques and may use their palms, arms, elbows, knees, and feet to vary the pressure and intensity of the treatment.*

DO IN: *A form of acupressure that is combined with breathing and exercise routines to stimulate the meridians and help prevent illness and disease.*

JIN SHEN (OR JIN SHIN): *A technique that specializes in prolonged pressure, sometimes lasting several minutes, applied to several specific points of the body.*

JIN SHEN DO: *A variation, among several, of Jin Shen. Each variation is identifiable by an extra word (in this case "Do") on the end. These differences appear so slight to the uninitiated as to be almost unimportant, but specialist skill in the subtleties is necessary for the therapy to be effective.*

SHEN TAO: *A variation used within Traditional Chinese Medicine that is similar to some of the gentler manipulative techniques. It can be likened to a form of healing that is achieved by the "laying-on-of-hands."*

ACUPRESSURE POINTS FOR PAIN RELIEF

Find out more

Massage	56
Acupuncture	68
Reflexology	74

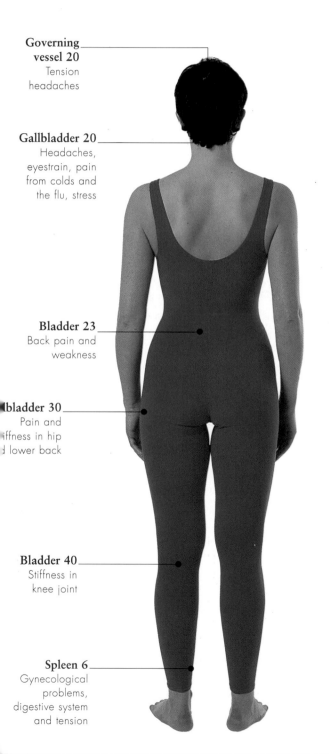

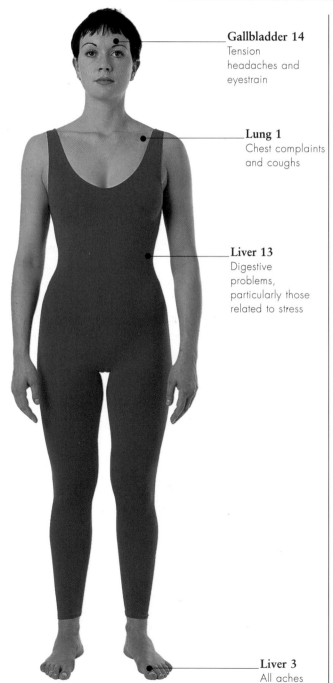

Governing vessel 20
Tension headaches

Gallbladder 20
Headaches, eyestrain, pain from colds and the flu, stress

Bladder 23
Back pain and weakness

bladder 30
Pain and iffness in hip d lower back

Bladder 40
Stiffness in knee joint

Spleen 6
Gynecological problems, digestive system and tension

Gallbladder 14
Tension headaches and eyestrain

Lung 1
Chest complaints and coughs

Liver 13
Digestive problems, particularly those related to stress

Liver 3
All aches and pains

Yoga

*I*ndian spiritual teachers developed this system of spiritual, *mental, and physical exercises over thousands of years. There are several different branches of yoga and many people can benefit from practices that range from quiet meditation to strenuous physical workouts.*

Yoga is effective in calming the mind and aiding relaxation. It also helps promote joint suppleness and muscle flexibility.

Yoga is more correctly known as a spiritual art—that is, it was originally devised to develop spiritual and physical awareness. It works through meditation, visualization, breathing exercises, and physical postures, all promoting a total attention to each moment of meditation or movement of the body.

In the West, the physical movements of Hatha yoga, in which the body is gently stretched into positions called *asanas*, is the most commonly practiced. But correct breathing and a mind emptied of other concerns are essential to each of these positions.

The yoga positions generally involve either stretching, twisting, or curling up the body. The alternate movements promote circulation, stimulate the functioning of the internal organs, and increase the flexibility of the body.

Yoga for pain relief

Yoga can also provide effective relief for many types of pain, particularly pain which results from muscular tension, such as menstrual cramps or tension headaches. It can relieve many digestive problems. Some positions can be used to loosen up restricted mobility caused by accident, injury, or inflammation of muscles, nerves, and joints and can be used for conditions such as back pain and arthritis. The *asanas* can also usefully correct distortions in body posture caused by working conditions. As our bodies age, they become used to simply sitting or standing and less able to bend and stretch. Yoga enables the aging body to loosen up and this improves the circulation of body fluids, the supply of nutrients to all parts of the body, and muscle tone, not only in the limbs but internally also.

At first, yoga should be practiced under supervision. People with heart or blood pressure problems should not practice certain positions and patients with any sort of chronic pain should consult their medical practitioner as well. However, the gentle approach to the positions generally allows each person to judge their own capacity and to increase it slowly.

Psychological benefits

Yoga promotes physical mobility and can have profound psychological benefits as well. Improvements in flexibility and circulation can help lift depression and the practice of awareness can help people who are under stress. The posture and tone of the body are known to induce emotional well-being.

In order to learn yoga it is best to find a good instructor, instead of using a book or a video, because the instructor will be able to supervise your movements and breathing. Today, yoga is so popular and widespread that it is easy to find supervised classes almost anywhere.

BASIC POSTURES

The aim of the yoga postures on this page is to promote and maintain the natural forward, backward, sideways, and twisting flexibility of the back. They are important exercises because keeping the back flexible is vital for full health and vitality.

Sideways bend

1 *Stand upright, with your legs wide apart, feet parallel, and arms down. Your palms should be against your thighs.*

2 *Breathe in slowly at the same time as you lift one arm straight up, the palm of the hand facing inward, until your arm touches the side of your head. Holding your breath, stretch your arm up as high you can, lifting your shoulder.*

3 *As you breathe out, bend slowly to one side, sliding your lower arm down your leg, until the upper arm is*

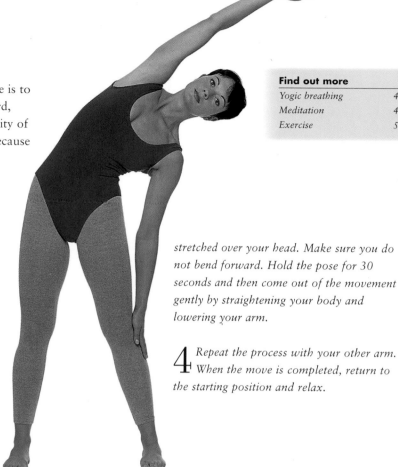

Find out more	
Yogic breathing	42
Meditation	48
Exercise	52

stretched over your head. Make sure you do not bend forward. Hold the pose for 30 seconds and then come out of the movement gently by straightening your body and lowering your arm.

4 *Repeat the process with your other arm. When the move is completed, return to the starting position and relax.*

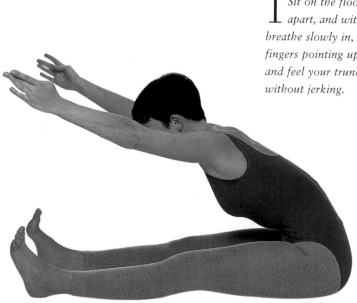

Back body stretch

1 *Sit on the floor with your legs straight out in front of you, slightly apart, and with your arms by your side. Breathe out. As you breathe slowly in, raise your arms so that they are vertical, with your fingers pointing upward. Stretch up as high as you can with your arms and feel your trunk lift as you do so. Do this slowly and deliberately, without jerking.*

2 *Breathe slowly out and, still maintaining the stretch, bring your arms slowly forward and down until they reach the furthest point on the legs that feels comfortable.*

3 *Holding the part you can reach, and still keeping the stretch, lower your head between your arms. Remain, breathing normally, for at least 30 seconds. Release and, as you breathe in, bring your body upright until your back is straight. Lie back and relax.*

How to breathe the yogic way

Breathing correctly is central to the practice of yoga. Indian yogis believe that through breathing we allow energy to enter the body and, in becoming fully aware of that breathing, we are being attentive to the life force. Mindfulness of breathing can provide help for respiratory problems.

One branch of yoga (*pranayama*) concentrates on awareness of the breath and on types of exercises with the breath. Some exercises emphasize deep, slow breaths, others the rapid, noisy expulsion of breath. These exercises have many benefits: they can contribute to meditation, as the awareness of breathing produces mental stillness. They can also help with respiratory conditions, such as asthma and bronchitis and relieve sinusitis. The tendency to fight for breath in asthma can be alleviated by the practice of yogic breathing. It will promote the supply of oxgen to the body and combat the bad effects of shallow breathing.

To breathe properly, you must use the diaphragm (the large dome of muscle that sits under the lungs) to push up on the lungs to empty and fill them properly. This is done by "abdominal breathing"— that is, breathing with your abdomen rather than your chest. Puffing your chest out is known as "thoracic breathing" and does not allow sufficient oxygen to get into the bloodstream.

The exercises below promote abdominal breathing. They should be done three times a day preferably first thing in the morning and last thing at night before going to bed.

Exercise for the lungs
• Lie flat on your back (on the floor or your bed is best).
• Bend your knees up so that your back is flat and touching the floor.
• Relax all your muscles as much as you can (it sometimes helps to have your eyes closed for this).
• Place one hand on your stomach to check that you are moving your stomach in and out rather than your chest and breathe in to a count of one and out to a count of one.
• Breathe in to a count of two and out to a count of two.
• Continue breathing in and out to longer and longer counts, up to seven or eight.
• Repeat the exercise for about 15 minutes and then relax.

Diaphragmatic breathing
• Make sure that your back is straight by lying flat or by standing up straight, whichever is the more comfortable.
• Slowly take in a deep breath, filling your lungs as much as possible.
• Tighten your stomach muscles, pulling them as flat as you can.
• Still holding your stomach muscles, breathe out so that you empty your lungs as completely as possible.
• Hold that position for one second and then release.
• Concentrate on breathing with your stomach, rather than your chest and shoulders. Allow your breathing to be as unforced and as natural as possible. It may take some time to develop a routine that comes without concentrating hard.
• Repeat the whole exercise for about 15 minutes and then relax.

T'ai chi

This ancient form of movement originated in China and is still so popular there that a common sight every morning in most major parks and public places is dozens, and sometimes hundreds, of people going through their daily t'ai chi routines. Like yoga, t'ai chi has spread to the West and is now widely practiced in many countries.

The essence of t'ai chi, which grew out of an even earlier Chinese system called qigong (pronounced "chi kung"), is the slow and graceful style of its movements. It has been aptly described as meditation in motion.

The aim of t'ai chi is to develop *chi* (life force) within the body as an antidote to aging and to encourage spiritual enlightenment. As with yoga, t'ai chi is also used to promote healing and maintain health.

T'ai chi provides both physical and psychological benefits, and is especially effective in releasing physical and psychological tensions.

GREETING THE DAWN

This is a simple and effective routine that takes about 5–10 minutes to carry out and is best done first thing in the morning. Each slow and graceful movement should flow into the next. Concentrate on balance and breathing and try to visualize each stage as you do it.

First movement: The mountain
Stand with your legs apart and slightly bent and your arms by your side. Try to feel as if you are "containing" the weight of your body in your loins (the source of qi in Chinese philosophy).

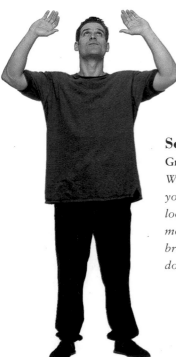

Second movement:
Greeting the dawn
Welcome the dawn by raising your arms in salute to the sky, looking upward. Hold for a moment and then slowly bring your arms around and down to your side.

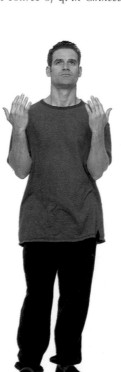

Third movement:
Acknowledging the past
Step back with one leg and salute the past by bringing both arms up and turning the palms of your hands so they face backward. ▶

T'ai chi

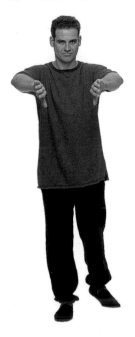

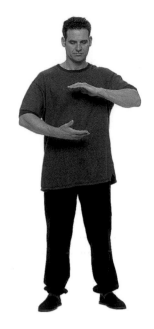

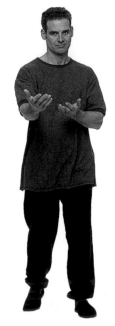

Fourth movement:
Drawing the curtains
Keeping the same position as in the third movement, transfer your weight to your front foot by rocking forward. Draw back an imaginary set of curtains with your hands.

Fifth movement:
Opening up to heaven and earth
Bring your back leg forward so you are now in an upright position. Using your arms and hands, imagine you are "drawing in" energy (qi) from the sky and ground and mixing it together at the level of your solar plexus.

Sixth movement:
Giving the energy away
Lean forward and, moving your hands and arms forward, "give the energy away" by visualizing it as being fire.

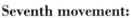

Seventh movement:
Receiving the rain
Lean back and "receive the rain" by drawing your hands down your body and visualizing the sensation of this as raindrops falling on you.

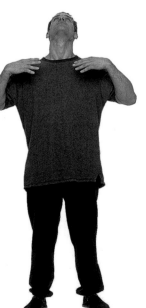

Eighth movement:
Checking out the universe
Move your legs with slow, deliberate, and balanced steps, as if you were a flexible, moving tree. Walk slowly around in a circle, "sensing" your surroundings with your hands.

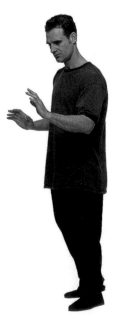

Ninth movement:
Gathering in the elements
Stand with your body centered. Using your right and left hands alternately, imagine you are gathering in the elements by scooping them up from either side.

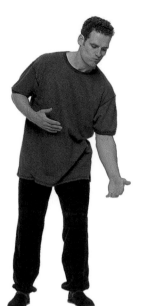

Tenth movement:
Returning the elements
Imagine you are giving everything you have gathered back to Creation by dropping your hands down and then throwing them up from the top of your head, as if you were throwing the energy from off your head.

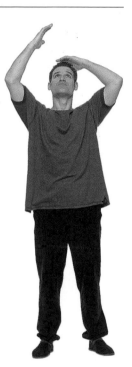

Eleventh movement:
Recovering the energy
Bend forward and, with both hands, imagine you are scooping up the energy from the ground.

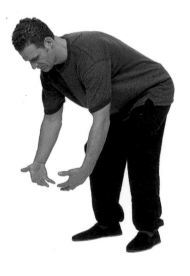

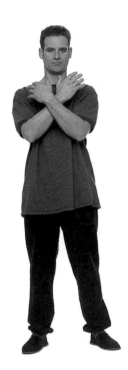

Twelfth movement:
Embracing the tiger
Bring your arms up and cross them in front of your chest, as if embracing.

Thirteenth movement:
Return to the mountain
Come to rest by placing your legs apart with your knees slightly bent, sensing the "weight" in your loins. Bend your arms at the elbows with your hands facing upward. Feel alive but at rest.

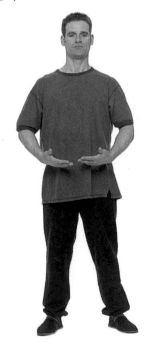

Self-help psychotherapies

Self-hypnosis, meditation, and visualization are techniques for inducing positive mental and psychological states. They can be used as a way of relaxing or to combat specific problems.

Self-help tapes can be an extremely effective way of calming the mind and "indoctrinating" it with positive thought patterns.

The techniques described below all work by the mind suggesting to itself certain mental states, usually using repetition of key phrases or images. People have used these techniques to combat addictions such as smoking, or eating disorders, or to contain pain.

Self-hypnosis

The Frenchman Emile Coué invented the term autosuggestion more than a century ago. Coué believed that repeating positive statements to yourself would change negative thought patterns into positive ones and he coined the famous phrase "Every day, in every way, I am getting better and better."

Self-hypnosis uses the power of the subconscious mind to persuade the conscious mind of something. People vary widely in how open to suggestion they are but, for some, it can be used effectively to alleviate chronic pain or combat psychological disorders, such as depression. Usually, patients will need to be shown how to do self-hypnosis but can then continue sessions by themselves.

Videos, audiotapes, and CDs are now available that offer self-hypnosis for a variety of mental and emotional problems. The results vary according to how an individual responds to a particular program.

Affirmations

The American healer Louise Hay invented a more modern version of self-hypnosis called affirmations in which the patient makes positive statements about himself or herself to counteract harmful negative thought patterns. Examples of Louise Hay affirmations are the following, which are best performed looking at yourself in a mirror:

• I am calm and confident.
• I love and approve of myself.
• I am the power and authority in my life and no one else is.
• I am filled with healing power.

Relaxation

Try the following relaxation technique to calm the nerves and release muscle tension throughout the whole body.

Lie comfortably on your back. Breathe slowly through your nose, as if you are sucking the air down into your abdomen. Point your toes and push them down as far as you can. After a few seconds, relax the toes. Repeat with your ankles. Then, tensing your muscles one by one, continue up your body until you reach your head. When you tense a particular muscle, focus your whole mind on it, feeling how strained it is. When you relax it, feel how heavy and relaxed it is.

BIOFEEDBACK THERAPY

In biofeedback therapy, fine electrodes, held either in the hand or connected to a band tied around your head, monitor your body's metabolism in terms of heartbeat, blood pressure, brain waves, and blood chemistry. With the help of a therapist, you can learn to control your metabolism by observing the meters and correcting their movements. You can thus induce a state of relaxation or control nausea or pain.

Biofeedback was developed during the U.S. space program in the 1960s when it was used by scientists at the NASA space center to teach astronauts how to control motion sickness.

Since then, people have been taught to regulate their blood pressure and heartbeat and, by controlling the side effects of pain, like sweating and accelerated pulse rate, can to some extent control the pain itself. By breaking down the effects of tension or pain into simple visible pointers, it appears to be easier for the mind to take control.

Biofeedback therapy is now well established, particularly in the United States, as a safe, gentle, and very effective way of promoting relaxation.

Since its introduction, biofeedback technology has developed considerably and it now includes a wide range of devices, varying in price and sophistication. Units range from simple hand-held battery-operated models for use at home to reclining armchairs linked to high-tech computer monitors, which are used by therapists at specialist centers.

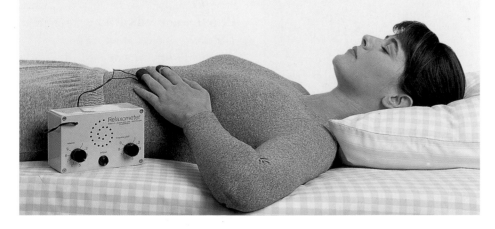

Meditation

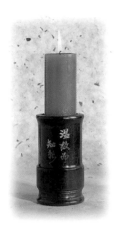

An object such as a fragrant lit candle may help you to concentrate by holding your attention, yet demanding nothing of you.

T*he mind can have a positive effect on the body if it can be freed from anxiety and emotional turmoil. Meditation can be used to calm the mind and put things in perspective. By accessing a deep level of consciousness, a person who practices meditation regularly can develop the ability to transcend pain.*

There are different levels of meditation which can be accessed. But, if the mind and body can become deeply relaxed, then beneficial effects will be experienced both for psychological states of tension and anxiety and for those physical disorders that seem to be especially related to stress.

Such disorders include hypertension, asthma, irritable bowel syndrome, and some skin conditions, which also seem to be caused by stress. Meditation works by inducing a state of deep relaxation but also by an increased awareness of and sensitivity to the normally unconscious body functions. Thus, such functions as body heat and heartbeat can be brought under conscious control.

Meditation induces a strong sense of peace and tranquillity, which many enjoy regardless of its therapeutic value. Research in Holland has shown that, when practiced regularly, transcendental meditation lowers blood pressure. As a result, health insurance premiums there were reduced for those who regularly practiced transcendental meditation.

Types of meditation

A wide variety of meditation techniques has been promoted in recent years, many by religious organizations making highly elaborate claims. Perhaps the most famous of these is transcendental meditation (TM). But there is, or should be, nothing mystical or mysterious about meditation. An example of an effective Western version of meditation without ritual is autogenic training (see Visualization, page 50).

Practicing meditation

The effects of meditation are not immediate but long-term meditators claim dramatic increases in energy, stamina, and resistance to ill health, as well as beneficial effects in the control of pain. For meditation to be successful, however, it must be practiced regularly.

Anyone can meditate but it takes practice to do it effectively, which is why it is best to be shown how to do it by an experienced teacher.

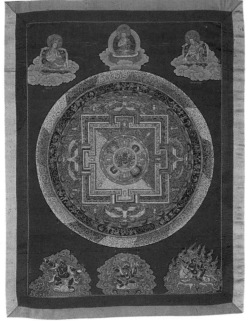

Focusing on a mandala, the oriental map symbolizing the universe, is often beneficial to meditation. The word mandala derives from the Sanksrit for circle, and most mandalas feature circular designs.

HOW TO MEDITATE

The aim of meditation is to relax the body and then the mind so that you can achieve a state of altered consciousness. It can be difficult at first but it becomes easier with practice. Ideally, you should meditate for about 30 minutes, both morning and the evening. You may find it easier if you develop the habit of meditating at a particular time so that it becomes part of your daily routine.

• Wear loose comfortable clothing that is not in the least restrictive.

• Choose somewhere quiet, warm but not hot, and well ventilated, where you will not be disturbed.

• Sit upright in a comfortable and well-supported position (if you lie down you could fall asleep and lose the whole point of the exercise). Let your shoulders relax, but try to keep your back straight. Rest your hands on your lap.

• Close your eyes or, if this makes you feel sleepy, try fixing your gaze on a single, simple object such as a lighted candle or a stone. The idea is to remain mentally alert yet relaxed.

• Breathe through the nose rather

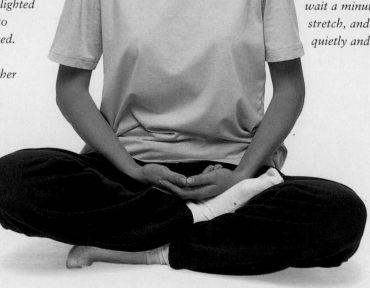

than the mouth. Breathe deeply but gently using the diaphragm muscle, rather than the chest.

• Repeat, silently or aloud, a single word or phrase over and over again. This is called a mantra in the Indian tradition and is similar to a chant. It does not really matter what the word is as long as the sound is pleasing and your mind becomes focused on it to the exclusion of everything else.

• Do not worry about stray thoughts that flit through your mind or how well you may or may not be doing. Instead, adopt a let-it-all-happen approach. Experienced meditators say, "don't push the river, let it flow by itself."

• Try to retain your concentration for at least half an hour. When you are ready to stop, open your eyes, wait a minute, then stretch, and get up quietly and slowly.

Visualization

The power of the imagination can be harnessed to help the body. It has been used effectively in the treatment of disorders as mild as coughing and as serious as cancer.

These exercises work in a similar manner to autosuggestion or some stages of meditation. A particular state of mind is induced, which may then have beneficial effects on the body. Cancer sufferers are encouraged to imagine an army of healthy cells attacking and destroying all the cancer cells in their body and replacing them with fresh, undamaged cells.

The results vary depending very much on the personality of the patient. The technique works best for people with good imaginations or for those who are able to allow their minds to express themselves freely. Perhaps for this reason children and young people tend to have more success than older adults, although anyone can achieve good results if they allow their minds such freedom.

In visualization, as in other techniques, such as relaxation and guided imagery, you can imagine yourself to be part of a tranquil, agreeable scene.

Pain visualization exercise

Before you start, get comfortable and relax. Breathe easily and let your mind settle. Whether the pain is physical or psychological, you should try and get a sense of it and describe what it feels like to you, or what it looks like. Is it throbbing, sharp or dull? Is it small, wide, or large? Is it light or heavy?

Having identified it as precisely as possible, the next step is to change it by imagining something appropriate in your mind's eye. For example, a heavy, wide, dull pain might be seen as a large rock pressing down on that part of you and a sharp, thin, light pain as a needle sticking into you.

Imagine yourself lifting that rock off you with ease, or being able to repel the

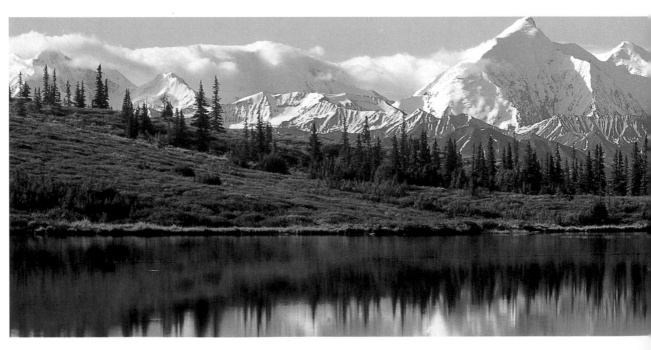

sharp pain because you are wearing thick armor.

Next, try to imagine you are somewhere where you feel happy and content. Gradually become part of the scene. See yourself as fit and well, totally pain-free, and with a positive outlook on life.

AUTOGENIC TRAINING

Autogenic training was developed by Dr. Johannes Schultz, a German psychiatrist and hypnotist. He noticed that the physiological effects of hypnosis, such as sensations of body warmth and relaxation of the muscles, could be induced by the patients themselves and were associated with release from stress and pain. The system he developed is related to both meditation (it is often called Western meditation), self-hypnosis, and yoga.

Students are taught how to do the exercises in one of three positions: lying, sitting in an armchair, or sitting in an upright chair, to allow them to do the exercises anywhere. Ideally, the exercises should be done three times a day after eating.

Autogenic training uses six standard exercises that involve directing your attention inwardly and focusing your mind:
- *sensations of heaviness in your body*
- *warmth in your arms and legs*
- *the calmness and regularity of your heart beat*
- *your easy and natural breathing*
- *warmth in your abdomen*
- *coolness in your head.*

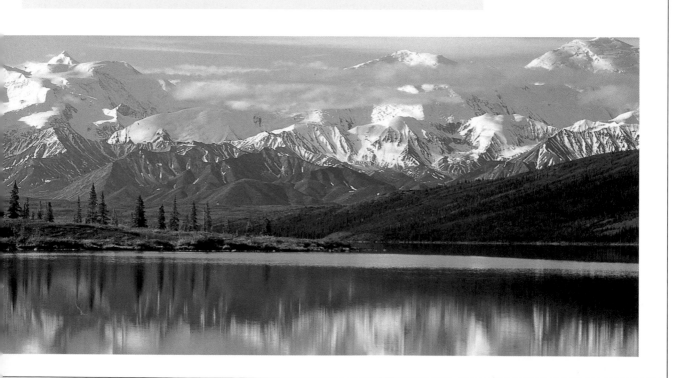

Exercise

R egular exercise will help to keep the body's functions in good condition and this will contribute to a feeling of physical and mental well-being.

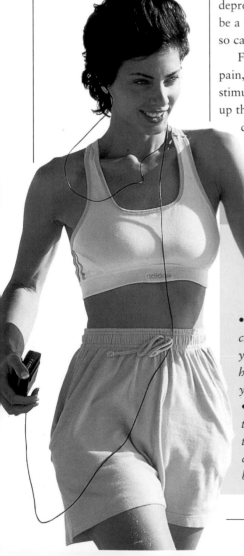

Running provides an excellent cardiovascular workout for the body and helps keep muscles and joints in good shape.

When the body has greater than usual demands made of it, many of its functions are stimulated by an increase in the blood and oxygen supply and this has wide-ranging effects on the feeling of general tone and well-being. The heart muscle is strengthened and the lungs breathe more deeply.

The increase in physical tone can have profound effects on mental pain, such as depression or anxiety. Exercise can also be a nonverbal method of expression and so can help to release pent-up emotions.

For people who are suffering physical pain, gentle exercise is recommended to stimulate the body's functions and loosen up the limbs, especially for inflammatory diseases such as arthritis and musculoskeletal problems.

How to exercise

The digestive system is one function that is inhibited by exercise, which is why you should not do vigorous exercise immediately after a meal.

Exercise should be suited to your physical state and you should consult your medical practitioner on what is best for you. The best forms of exercise for pain sufferers are swimming, walking, or gentle jogging, but even if you cannot do any of these, some gentle exercise may be possible.

To feel a real benefit from exercise, you need to have a 20-minute session three or four times a week. Fitness cannot be stored so regular exercise is essential. The beneficial effects of exercise wear off after 24 hours, so you should resolve to exercise regularly throughout your life.

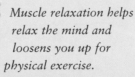

RELAXATION EXERCISE

Muscle relaxation helps relax the mind and loosens you up for physical exercise.

• *Sit in a comfortable position on a chair. Starting with your feet, wiggle your toes. Squeeze your feet with your hands for a moment and then rotate your ankles.*

• *Progressing up the legs, squeeze or tense your calves, knees, and thighs in turn before relaxing. At each stage be conscious of the difference in feeling before and after.*

• *Next, clench your buttocks, hold for a few seconds, and then relax.*

• *Slowly breathe in and tighten the stomach muscles. Hold for a few moments and then release as you slowly breathe out.*

• *Many people hold tension in their shoulders. To release it, hunch your shoulders up. Hold for a few moments and then release, making sure you allow the tension to leave the muscles.*

• *Screw up your face and stretch your jaw. Release.*

• *Gently stretch your body and relax.*

Jumping jacks

Begin with feet together and arms hanging loosely by your sides. Jump so that you land with your feet a little more than hip-width apart. At the same time swing your arms up so your hands cross above your head. Jump back to the start position and repeat five times.

Jogging

Jog gently in place for five minutes, keeping your head erect and back straight.

Find out more	
Musculoskeletal system	18
Yoga	40
Physiotherapy	82

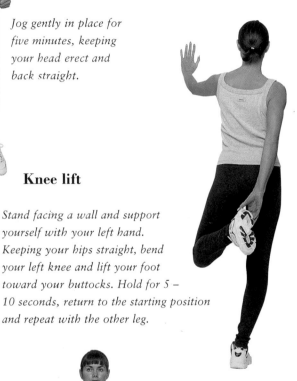

Forward lunge

Stand with hands on hips. Breathe in as you step forward with your right foot, leaving your left foot where it is. Hold your breath and bend your right knee to an angle of 90 degrees. Hold for 8 – 10 seconds, then repeat with the left leg. Repeat five times.

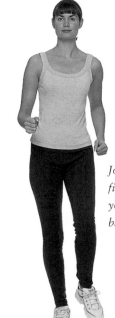

Knee lift

Stand facing a wall and support yourself with your left hand. Keeping your hips straight, bend your left knee and lift your foot toward your buttocks. Hold for 5 – 10 seconds, return to the starting position and repeat with the other leg.

Back stretch

Kneel with your hands on the floor in front of you. Gently push your hands away from you as far as they will go, leaning forward to bring your body closer to the floor. Hold for 8 – 10 seconds, slowly return to the start position, and repeat 5 – 10 times.

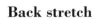

Waist twist

Stretch your arms out in front of you at shoulder height. Bend your right elbow and push it backward, turning your upper body to the right as far as it will go without straining. Hold for 1 – 2 seconds, slowly return to the start position and repeat on the other side. Repeat the sequence 5 – 10 times.

Creative arts therapies

D*ance, painting, music, drama, and other forms of creative activity can be used to explore and express psychological states and emotions in a nonverbal way. By releasing stress and blocked emotions, corresponding physical pain is alleviated.*

People of all ages and abilities can use creative arts as a therapeutic means of expressing psychological problems, such as depression, phobias, obsessions, and addictions. They are especially valuable for those who have difficulty expressing themselves in words.

The creative arts have been shown to be a very potent tool for communication, not only with others, but also within the self, and it is the nonverbal aspect that is the significant part of this growing form of psychotherapy.

All these therapies can be practiced at home without any training. However, working with a trained therapist can encourage you to explore your emotions and find an effective means of expression.

Music therapy

Creating sound either with the voice or musical instruments can allow free expression of inner feelings and emotions that might not otherwise find an outlet. Simply listening to music that stirs the feelings can provide valuable emotional freedom. Music therapy can also help speech disorders, such as stammering, and is used with deaf people to give them some feeling of sound and rhythm.

Dance therapy

Physical movements allow some people to draw out and express inner feelings that may not be easy to talk about. Based on the work of the 1920s pioneer, Rudolf von Laban, dance therapy is most effective when done in groups under the guidance of a trained therapist, but can be done alone at home. Dancing can also be a gentle way of moving the body for sufferers from arthritic pain or people recovering the use of limbs or muscles after accidents.

Art therapy

Free inner expression can be released through art. Painting, modeling, or sculpting are common forms of expression but any medium can be used, depending on what you prefer. In all cases, freely expressing the innermost

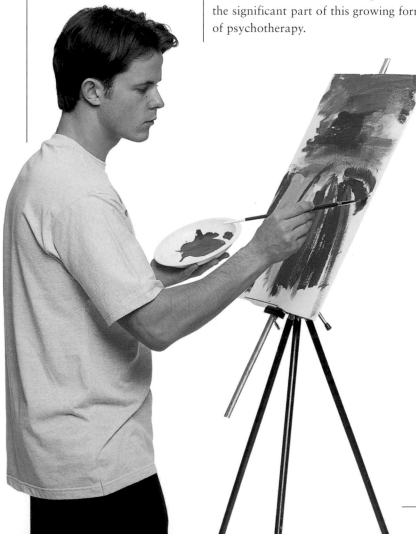

Abstract painting is a form of self-expression that allows the mind to work in an unrestricted, free-form manner.

feelings is the aim of the therapy and the artistic standard of the work or the competence of the artist is unimportant.

Painting can be used as a physical form of visualization or as a way of giving vent to inner feelings, for example, anger, joy, or grief. The painting may be a specific representation of an emotion—a self-portrait of a happy or unhappy face, for example, but therapists try to encourage a more abstract or surreal approach so that the painter is not distracted by technique. Often, the images that emerge from the inner mind can be related to childhood events or traumas and interpretation can help toward dealing with them.

The physical act of splashing paint onto a canvas or throwing and molding clay with your hands provides the release. A trained therapist can help provide insights into problems and encourage healing by watching how a person works and exploring the process with them.

Drama therapy

The therapeutic uses of role enactment were formulated first in Europe and then in the United States during the 1920s by Jacob Moreno. Closely allied to psychodrama, drama therapy is now well established and widely practiced.

Drama therapy encourages you to be someone or something else so that you can gain an insight into your own problems viewed from a different perspective. This also allows you to experiment with various possible solutions. By acting out imaginary situations in a group you may uncover hidden or repressed feelings. At home, drama therapy can be used in the same way, although the insights gained may be less revealing.

Sand play therapy

By playing with miniature toys in the "world" of the sand tray, the past, present, or future can be worked through therapeutically with the help of a trained therapist. This medium is widely used to help children express themselves but adults can also find it a very effective outlet for emotional problems.

Find out more

Self-help psychotherapies	46
Psychotherapy	76
Treatments for emotional pain	92

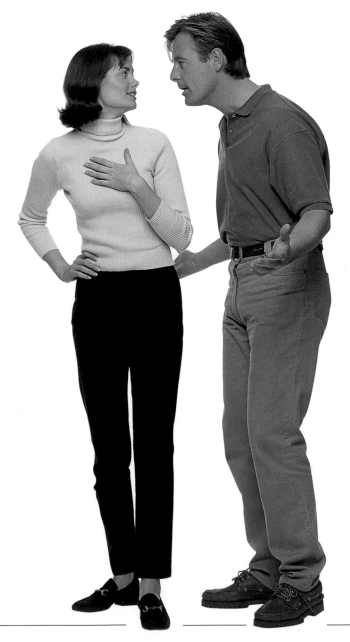

Drama therapy uses role playing to allow for the safe exploration of emotional problems.

Massage

R*ubbing a painful spot is probably the most instinctive remedy. More extensive massage can be helpful for many conditions from stress to different types of pain.*

Whether to relax aching muscles and joints or as a treatment for various disorders, massage is increasingly used in a large number of hospitals and nursing clinics, particularly for providing relief from chronic pain. It can also be very enjoyable practiced with a spouse. The techniques are easy to learn, and both partners can benefit from the shared intimacy and the extra time spent together.

Key areas of the body, which can become very tense and stiff and even misaligned from stress, are the neck, shoulders, and the back, and these areas can benefit greatly from massage.

A massage can provide short-term relief from chronic pain for cancer patients, ease stiff joints, or prevent tension headaches or migraines.

Massage styles

There are many variations of massage techniques, from the firm pressures used in Swedish massage to the gentle soothing approach, which has more in common with the soft tissue manipulation used by some osteopaths or hands-on healers.

The effectiveness of massage is due to its ability to help stimulate the flow of blood around the body and relax tight nerves and muscles. It also provides the equally important psychological benefit of feeling "cared for."

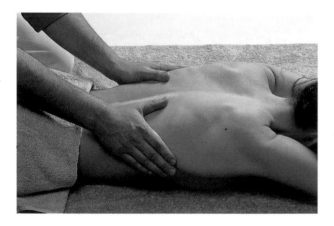

Stroking (effleurage)

This is the most basic massage technique and is used to start and end the massage. Stroking should last at least half an hour for best results. Position your hands flat and pointing up the body. Slide them over the back, making the movements long and slow. Use more pressure on the upward strokes than on those going downward.

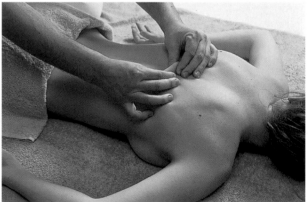

Kneading (petrissage)

This technique uses the fingers and thumbs to squeeze and roll the surface tissues of the skin against the tissues beneath, similar to kneading dough. It is used on fleshier areas, such as the hips and thighs, to loosen muscle stiffness, improve circulation, and break down fatty deposits so they can be eliminated more easily.

PERFORMING A MASSAGE

Find out more

Aromatherapy	36
Acupressure	38
Physiotherapy	82

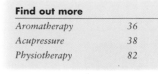

The person being massaged should lie down on a comfortable but firm surface in a warm room. Have a couple of large towels handy to keep them warm. To allow the hands to slide easily over the skin, use a neutral oil. These are widely available, especially in health outlets and pharmacies. Aromatherapy oils can be used with great effect

(see Aromatherapy massage, page 36).

The techniques shown here are those used by professionals. They are easy to learn and perform and can be applied to any age group of either sex, including children and babies.

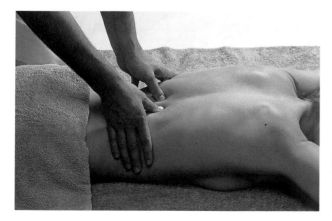

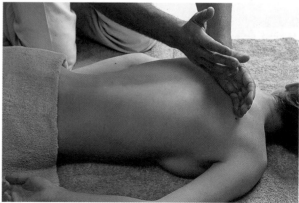

Friction (frottage)

This is a variation on kneading and has a similar effect. Use the fingers, thumbs, or heel of the hand to make small, circular movements on the skin. Circling can be used where you feel a particular tension or "knot." To relax a muscle, press gently, slowly circling the area and increasing the pressure when you feel a response.

Percussion (tapotement)

Percussion uses the hands to stimulate the circulation and encourage the breakdown of tension and stiffness. This technique uses a "hacking" movement with the sides of the fingers. Because of its relatively strong action, treatment is sometimes confined to the buttocks, thighs, and calves. It is not recommended for use on ultrasensitive people.

CHAPTER TWO

Massage aids

A variety of massage devices can be used to supplement or replace the hands. They can be obtained through health stores, pharmacies, sports retailers, and mail-order companies and are used in many pain clinics.

Some people find that, when massaging themselves, a massage aid is more effective than a hand massage alone. Using a tool may make it easier to reach the area or may demand less physical effort from the patient. Massage aids vary from the simple shaped wooden tool with which you can knead the muscles to more sophisticated electrical devices. As with most therapies, treatment usually needs to be prolonged (for up to an hour) and regular (at least daily) for maximum effect.

At their best, massage aids can produce relief from pain that lasts for several hours, and sometimes days, after treatment.

The simplest aids are those that use balls or rollers attached to a handle. These are run over the body using different pressures. Often made of wood, these aids are available in a wide range of shapes and sizes and are relatively inexpensive to buy. Most people find them easy to use and find they have a very relaxing effect.

There are also various electrical massage aids that can help provide pain relief for a wide range of conditions (see opposite).

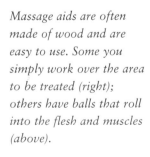

Massage aids are often made of wood and are easy to use. Some you simply work over the area to be treated (right); others have balls that roll into the flesh and muscles (above).

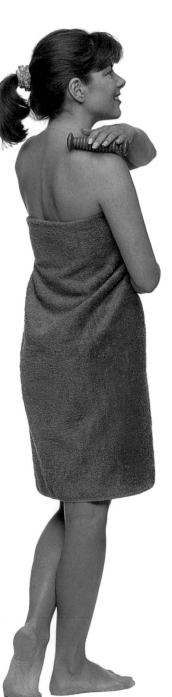

ELECTRICAL MASSAGE AIDS

A more sophisticated range of aids uses an electrical current, either from internal batteries or a main supply, to deliver stimulation via vibration, light, or sound. Some devices use a combination of stimuli, for example combining vibration effects with infrared light treatment. These treatments enable the patient to be more passive and can therefore be more relaxing, especially if the treament is to alleviate serious pain.

VIBRATION

Electrical vibrations can promote healing by stimulating blood flow to the affected area and by inhibiting pain messages from being sent to the brain.

The machines come in a variety of shapes and sizes, from basic inexpensive handheld devices to sophisticated and expensive reclining couches, chairs, and beds. Some vibrating recliners include heat treatment with essential oils, biofeedback, and ambient music.

Differently shaped and textured heads or "applicators" are fitted onto the handheld devices to suit the user's needs. These include "deep heat" devices that can also be used with essential oils for added effect; devices that mimic the hand movements of a massage therapist; and those that massage the acupressure points.

LIGHT

The use of infrared light is well known and widely used in both the orthodox and complementary treatment of pain. The rays produced by infrared light penetrate into soft tissues and warm them at a much deeper level and much more quickly than is possible in any other way. The treatment is useful both in emergency treatment for physical trauma and in the relief of chronic pain in conditions such as arthritis.

The therapy is painless and safe if used in accordance with the instructions. Unlike aids that require half an hour or more of treatment to be effective, infrared therapy can produce relief in as little as 5–10 minutes.

SOUND

Sound-wave therapy was first developed in the 1920s in Sweden but it is only in recent years that a handheld device has become available, offering a quick and easy method of self-help for pain relief.

The "intrasound" device works in much the same way as the electrical vibration devices but may penetrate to a deeper level. Low-level sound waves are sent through the tissues to stimulate blood flow and other metabolic processes at the site of the pain and accelerate the healing process of the body. The sound waves are generated by passing electricity through a crystal inside the metal head of the instrument. The treatment is both painless and soundless.

The device can be useful when damaged tissues are too tender to touch but it should be used with caution if the tissues are actually damaged. Results are variable but some pain sufferers claim it helps dramatically.

Herbal medicine

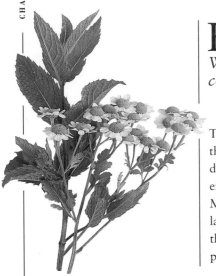

Herbalism is probably the oldest form of medical science and was almost the only effective form of medicine in the Western world until the 18th century. Today, in many poorer countries, it is still the predominant form of treatment.

The use of herbs is enjoying a revival in the West, perhaps because of growing disenchantment with the unpleasant side effects of many pharmaceutical drugs. Modern pharmaceutical medicine is largely derived from herbal medicine in that most modern medicines are based on plant products, but these drugs are now mostly synthesized rather than being extracted from plant material. This means that the drug is a pure concentrate without the other natural chemicals found in the herb or plant, which may all act together. Herbalists believe that these strong, synthetically produced chemicals may have various ill effects on the body,

HERB	EFFECTS	USES
ALOE VERA	Purgative (internal), soothing (external)	Used internally to increase menstrual flow; used externally for burns, bites, painful skin conditions. **Do not use if pregnant.**
ARNICA	Anti-inflammatory, wound healing	Bruises, sprains, rheumatic pain, phlebitis, general skin pain
CALENDULA	Anti-inflammatory, antifungal, astringent, wound healing	Skin inflammation, cuts, bruises, sprains, skin ulcers, burns, scalds, indigestion and digestive problems, ulcers, painful periods
CHAMOMILE	Antispasmodic, anti-inflammatory, painkiller, antiseptic, wound healing	Anxiety, insomnia, indigestion, gastritis, gas, dyspepsia, gingivitis, sore eyes, sore throat, phlegm and congestion, sinusitis, cuts, swelling from inflammation
CLOVE	Antiseptic, anesthetic, stimulant	Nausea, vomiting, gas, tooth and gum ache
CRAMP BARK (VIBURNUM)	Antispasmodic, sedative, astringent	Muscle pain and cramps, muscle spasms, menstrual pains and cramps, heavy periods
ECHINACEA	Antibiotic, immune-stimulant, anti-inflammatory, anti-allergenic	Bacterial and viral infections, the flu, laryngitis, tonsillitis, gingivitis, sores, cuts, boils, septicemia, cystitis
EUCALYPTUS	Decongestant, antiseptic	Respiratory illnesses, wounds, cuts
FEVERFEW	Anti-inflammatory, relaxant	Migraines, arthritis, tinnitus, dizziness, painful periods, weak periods
GARLIC	Antiseptic, antifungal, antiviral, antispasmodic, antimicrobial, hypotensive	Infections, digestive and respiratory pain (bronchitis, phlegm, colds, flu, asthma), ringworm, high blood pressure, arterial congestion

and in the end may be less effective. To distinguish what they offer from both native herbal remedies and synthetic drugs, modern herbalists tend to use terms such as "phytotherapy," and "botanical medicine," rather than "herbal medicine."

Oriental herbs from Traditional Chinese Medicine and the Ayurvedic medical tradition are now increasingly being adopted by Western herbalists, who have been drawing on the best of both European and North American traditions for some time.

Taking herbal remedies

Herbal remedies are available in tablet or capsule form from good pharmacies and health retail outlets and can be used as self-treatment for a wide range of minor health problems. For individual treatment for more serious conditions it is strongly advised that you see a qualified herbalist. Herbs are powerful drugs—and dangerous in untrained hands. To ensure you use the right herb in the right dosage without the risk of side effects, only go to herbalists who are fully qualified.

Find out more

Aromatherapy	36
Naturopathy	62
Homeopathy	70

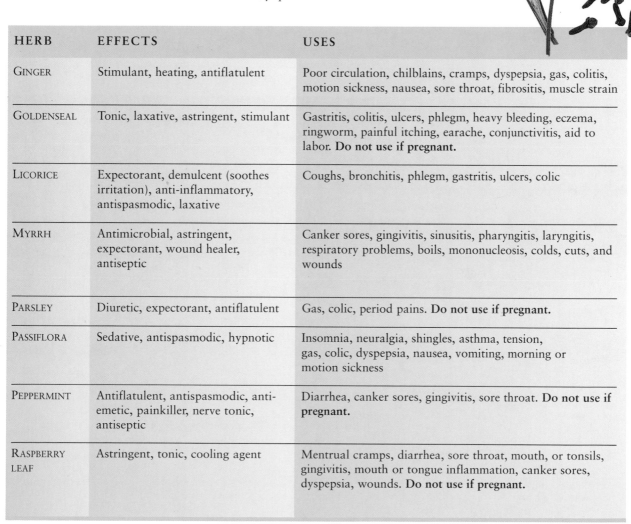

HERB	EFFECTS	USES
GINGER	Stimulant, heating, antiflatulent	Poor circulation, chilblains, cramps, dyspepsia, gas, colitis, motion sickness, nausea, sore throat, fibrositis, muscle strain
GOLDENSEAL	Tonic, laxative, astringent, stimulant	Gastritis, colitis, ulcers, phlegm, heavy bleeding, eczema, ringworm, painful itching, earache, conjunctivitis, aid to labor. **Do not use if pregnant.**
LICORICE	Expectorant, demulcent (soothes irritation), anti-inflammatory, antispasmodic, laxative	Coughs, bronchitis, phlegm, gastritis, ulcers, colic
MYRRH	Antimicrobial, astringent, expectorant, wound healer, antiseptic	Canker sores, gingivitis, sinusitis, pharyngitis, laryngitis, respiratory problems, boils, mononucleosis, colds, cuts, and wounds
PARSLEY	Diuretic, expectorant, antiflatulent	Gas, colic, period pains. **Do not use if pregnant.**
PASSIFLORA	Sedative, antispasmodic, hypnotic	Insomnia, neuralgia, shingles, asthma, tension, gas, colic, dyspepsia, nausea, vomiting, morning or motion sickness
PEPPERMINT	Antiflatulent, antispasmodic, anti-emetic, painkiller, nerve tonic, antiseptic	Diarrhea, canker sores, gingivitis, sore throat. **Do not use if pregnant.**
RASPBERRY LEAF	Astringent, tonic, cooling agent	Mentrual cramps, diarrhea, sore throat, mouth, or tonsils, gingivitis, mouth or tongue inflammation, canker sores, dyspepsia, wounds. **Do not use if pregnant.**

Naturopathy and hydrotherapy

A range of natural medicinal therapies is included in the general term naturopathy. One of the most important of these is hydrotherapy, also known as water therapy, an effective natural treatment for pain.

The use of water to treat pain dates back 2,500 years. After centuries of neglect hydrotherapy is now commonly used by practitioners of both orthodox and complementary medicine.

Hippocrates, the father of modern medicine in ancient Greece, was perhaps the first advocate of naturopathy. He believed that the body will cure itself provided it has only pure air and water, is kept clean, indulges only in healthy activities, and eats wholesome food.

This philosophy was revived in central Europe in the 19th century, by a new generation of pioneers including Benedict Lust in Germany. Modern naturopathy began when Henry Lindlahr and Benedict

Lust emigrated to the United States in the early years of the 20th century and the term "naturopathy" was coined in the United States by Lust.

Modern naturopathy

Naturopathy today is centered around the principle that the body's natural state is a healthy one and that the body will always tend toward a healthy state if it can. It is the aim of the practitioner and the patient, therefore, to enable the body to

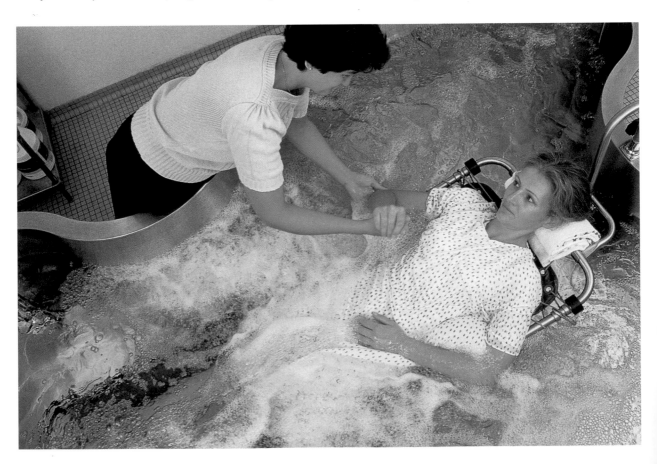

cure itself. Linked to this picture of the natural state of the body is the idea that disease itself is a natural phenomenon and that the symptoms of disease are often simply the result of the healing process. At the simplest level, excess mucus and sneezing are the way the body eliminates the cold-bearing virus.

Naturopathic therapies encapsulate most of the tenets of complementary medicine. Naturopaths treat the body and mind as a whole and will analyze the patient's whole lifestyle, including work and diet, before recommending therapies which may range from massage to homeopathic medicine. Rather than suppressing the symptoms of illness, naturopathic treatment encourages the symptoms to come out. The body is then stimulated to fight the symptoms and regain its proper balance.

Naturopaths routinely encourage brief fasting for simple infections such as the flu. They also pay careful attention to the health of the intestines because this is where nutrients are absorbed into the bloodstream. Toxins in the bowels can cause many digestive problems.

Special diets to clear the gut and eliminate the overgrowth of hostile yeasts and bacteria are also recommended. According to naturopaths, these contribute to toxicity, allergy, and poor immunity in the body.

Known as "nature cure" or "natural hygiene," this pure approach still survives among a few naturopaths who believe that it is even wrong to prescribe extra nutrients in the form of vitamin and mineral supplements. Naturopaths do not recommend self-help through nutritional therapy, particularly if it involves high doses of supplements, without receiving their advice and guidance first.

Naturopathy and other therapies

Modern naturopathy has extended its repertoire to include complementary therapies and many naturopaths are also practitioners in other therapies. Those trained at specialist colleges study herbalism, massage, homeopathy, manipulation, acupuncture, hypnotherapy, nutritional and dietary therapy, and hydrotherapy. In addition, they will refer patients to qualified practitioners in therapies such as chiropractic and osteopathy in order to achieve total health for their patients.

This wide-ranging approach is now the basis of modern naturopathy and it has become the standard training for those studying natural medicine at its broadest level.

Hydrotherapy

Modern hydrotherapy was developed by the 19th century Austrian physician Vincent Preissnitz. Hydrotherapy involves the therapeutic use of water in the form of swimming, douches, jet sprays, hot and cold baths, hot and cold compresses, showers, steam (Turkish) baths, and saunas. Some of these need the guidance of the naturopath or special facilities but some therapeutic techniques can be used at home by the patient.

HYDROTHERAPY FOR PAIN

Hydrotherapy is becoming increasingly popular as a treatment used in mainstream physiotherapy. It is particularly effective in stimulating circulation, relieving respiratory disorders, and alleviating muscle and joint pain after injury or in long-term conditions, such as arthritis. Hydrotherapy can be stimulating or soothing and can also be very effective in treating emotional and mental problems.

Bodywork techniques

Expert manipulation of the body, especially the bones and muscles of the spine, can help a range of persistent long-term, or chronic, problems. Chiropractic and osteopathy are the best known and most effective of these so-called bodywork therapies for pain relief.

Many elements of our lives produce distortions of our skeletal and muscular framework. Bad posture at work, repetitive one-sided actions, or carrying loads can all make for problems and pain. The group of therapies described here are some of the complementary therapies available.

Chiropractic

The aim of chiropractic is to restore health and balance by manipulation of the bones, muscles, and tissues of the body, particularly of the spine.

Developed by Canadian Daniel David Palmer at the end of the 19th century, chiropractic considers that the treatment

mainly affects the nerves of the body. This contrasts with osteopathy, which believes the blood supply is the determining factor.

Chiropractic is also generally more vigorous than osteopathy and its practitioners are somewhat more conventionally clinical in approach, including the use of X rays in diagnosis. Techniques vary from the high-velocity sudden thrusts used by some chiropractors to adjust joints to the relatively gentle slower movements which will coax bones and muscles into place.

Osteopathy

The word "osteopathy" means "bone treatment" but osteopathy aims to improve the overall structure of the body. Its practitioners claim that it can benefit almost any disorder, including pain, through the manipulation of the bones, muscles, and the soft tissues of the body.

Osteopathy was developed in the United States more than 100 years ago by Dr. Andrew Taylor Still, an army doctor. Today, it is so well established in the United States that its practitioners are

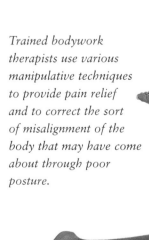

Trained bodywork therapists use various manipulative techniques to provide pain relief and to correct the sort of misalignment of the body that may have come about through poor posture.

all conventional doctors with extra training in manipulation.

Osteopaths concentrate on manipulating soft tissue rather than bones and will probe deeply to find areas of tension. Another technique is to use the passive movement of the patient's limbs to free up muscles and ligaments.

Cranial osteopathy

A further development of osteopathy is cranial osteopathy which, with its latest variant craniosacral therapy, claims to treat the whole body by using very gentle manipulation of the bones of the head and also, to some extent, the spine.

The bones of the skull protect the brain, which is insulated by a thin layer of fluid called the cerebrospinal fluid. The cerebrospinal fluid also protects the spinal cord within the spinal column. Cranial osteopaths believe that, if the passage of this fluid becomes blocked, physical or emotional disease occurs. By placing the hands lightly on the patient's head and using the softest pressure, the therapist aims to release these restrictions to restore balance and proper function.

Trigger-point therapy

Trigger-point therapy aims to relieve pain in the musculoskeletal system by concentrating on those points where the nerve cells that relay messages to the brain are connected to the muscle. These points are known as "trigger points." The neuromuscular spindle is the sensory receptor that controls stretch. Pain causes the spindle to tighten the muscle tissue. This puts strain on the connecting tissues and joints, increasing the pain.

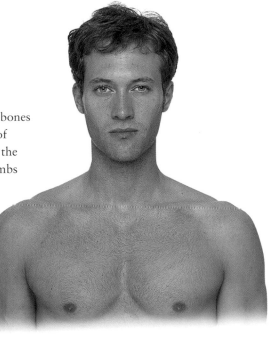

Find out more	
Musculoskeletal system	18
Massage	56
Physiotherapy	82

Osteopathy is best known as a treatment to repair structural misalignments in the body, especially in the spine, and to restore balance and improve posture. A consultation with an osteopath may also involve advice on diet and other lifestyle factors that may affect your pain.

Trigger-point therapy applies sustained pressure to the muscles to override the tensing effect of the pain messages and induce stretch in the muscles. Regular treatment aims to break the "pain–tension–pain" cycle and allow the muscles to relax and function well.

Visceral osteopathy

This technique manipulates and massages the viscera (soft organs of the abdomen) to improve their health and function. Typically, it is used to correct problems in the stomach, pancreas, and small and large intestines. The therapist applies a slow and controlled probing pressure to the organs to detect any malfunctions or abnormalities, such as lumps. These areas are then eased with gentle massage.

Myofascial release therapy

In this therapy strong and deep pressure is used on the muscular connective tissue (myofascial tissue) to loosen areas of tension in conditions such as neuralgia. The therapy can be painful and is similar in technique to Rolfing (see page 66). ▶

Bodywork techniques

In the latter part of the 20th century it has been increasingly recognized that mental and emotional factors can have an adverse effect on the musculoskeletal system. Unhappiness or stress will be translated into tight muscles and an unbalanced posture. This in turn may produce long-term pain and distorted musculature.

A number of techniques have been developed to improve on the physical manipulation of the body by taking these factors into account, and some of the principal ones are described below.

Rolfing

The German-born biochemist Ida Rolf developed this technique in the United States in the 1930s. She recognized that we can either meet the force of gravity in a harmonious spirit and allow our bodies to be balanced or we can fight gravity and thus produce tensions and misalignments in our bodies.

The essence of Rolfing is in "structural integration"—that is, strengthening and realigning the body through vigorous massage. Rolfing often uses the elbows and even the knees to dig deeply into muscle fascia (the tissue that binds muscle fibers together) to loosen and correct any misshaping of the body that may have developed over time through injury, trauma, and bad posture.

An improvement in posture will often also afford considerable relief to conditions like asthma and digestive problems, but some patients will find the Rolfing manipulation too uncomfortable.

THE ALEXANDER TECHNIQUE

This technique was developed early in the 20th century by Frederick Matthias Alexander, an Australian actor, when he found his career in jeopardy because of problems with voice production. By carefully studying himself in mirrors as he recited, he realized that the carriage of the head and neck are central to good posture.

Alexander believed that the development of the human race has robbed us of our instinctive knowledge of our physical selves and that work and sedentary lifestyles are to blame for bad posture.

The method must first be learned from a qualified teacher in 4 – 6 lessons but can then be used without instruction. The technique is a way of relearning how to use the body with maximum effect and minimum strain.

The technique has grown in popularity and is now widely used for overcoming muscle and joint problems, such as neck and back problems, and fibrositis. Those with circulation and breathing problems and recurrent headaches and migraines may also benefit from using the technique. Alexander technique is especially popular with musicians whose playing positions, sustained for many hours, produce distortions of the body.

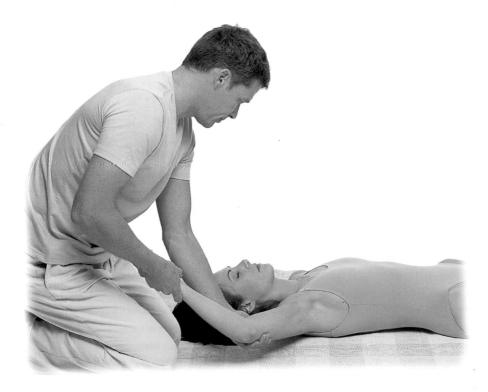

Hellerwork, in common with other bodywork techniques, aims to balance and realign the body through a combination of joint manipulation and massage.

Hellerwork, the Trager approach, and the Feldenkrais method

These therapies are said to be particularly effective for musculoskeletal problems, sciatica, and associated nerve pains, aches and pains due to headaches and migraines, stress, and asthma. The therapies use a combination of manipulation and movement.

Hellerwork and the Trager approach were developed in the United States in the 20th century (by Joseph Heller and Milton Trager) and both aim to reeducate the body to function correctly by encouraging the unconscious mind to adjust misalignments in the musculoskeletal system.

The Trager approach is said to be particularly effective for pain control and includes a system of "mentastics"—mental exercises that can be practiced at home.

Feldenkrais is also very similar, being described as "functional integration" and "awareness through movement." It was created by a Russian-born engineer, Moshe Feldenkrais, who emigrated to the United Kingdom in 1940.

Rosen method

This gentle manipulative technique is one of many which arose in the West Coast of United States in the latter part of the 20th century in the training of techniques such as Rolfing. The Rosen method combines physical movement and psychotherapeutic theories of mind–body interaction with breathing exercises and relaxation techniques. The method is, however, without formal structure and disciplines and therapists are taught more to act on their own intuition and experience than on training.

Acupuncture

The ancient Chinese developed the theory that the balance of the body can be treated by the insertion of very fine needles—so fine that most people hardly feel them being inserted —at points situated along the energy meridians of the body.

The Chinese believed that the body's energy, or *chi*, flows along energy lines or meridians. There are 12 main meridians, associated with particular organs, such as the lung meridian or the gallbladder meridian, and the 365 main acupuncture points are found along the meridians. Acupuncture at these points is thought to stimulate the flow of the energy. The technique originated more than 4,000 years ago, although the earliest books on the subject did not appear until 475 BC.

In Chinese philosophy disease is diagnosed by assessing the humors or elements in the body and illnesses are attributed to imbalances in wind, cold, damp, or heat.

A significant and growing number of physiotherapists and doctors use acupuncture largely for giving pain relief but also for treating addictions. Acupuncture is also used in some Western hospitals as an alternative to anesthetic.

Most orthodox doctors do not accept the theory of acupuncture but, because research has shown definite benefits, they have adopted a more clinical form of the therapy known as Western acupuncture. Often they prefer to use electro-acupuncture. This delivers a weak electric current via the needles for greater effect, especially on the points on the ear, which are believed to have the same meridians as the body (auricular therapy).

ACUPUNCTURE NEEDLES

Acupuncture needles come in a variety of shapes and sizes to suit different purposes. For use on the body they range from 0.25 inch to 2 inches (7 mm to 50 mm) in length. For auricular acupuncture, needles resembling press-studs are used, although ordinary needles can also be used on the ears. Special needles are used for blood-letting and general body "tapping."

Archaeological evidence indicates that early Chinese practitioners used needles made from bone, bamboo, and even sharp stones. Today, they are made of tensile-strength metal, usually stainless steel. Better quality needles are plated with the neutral metals of gold or silver. In moxibustion, a needle with a copper-coiled handle is used to help conduct the heat given off by the moxa down to the point where the needle is inserted into the body. In the Orient, needles are often reused but in the West responsible practitioners use sterile "one-use" needles to avoid transmitting serious infections, such as HIV.

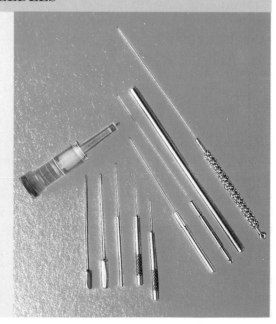

TRADITIONAL CHINESE MEDICINE

Find out more

| Acupressure | 38 |
| TCM and eczema | 97 |

Acupuncture, auricular acupuncture, moxibustion, cupping, and Chinese herbal medicine are all part of Traditional Chinese Medicine (TCM), an ancient and widely used system of diagnosing and treating disease. Western practitioners of TCM tend to concentrate solely on the use of acupuncture and moxibustion.

The number of herbs used in Chinese medicine is vast and many are extremely strong. For this reason, practitioners in the West are usually Chinese, as few Western practitioners have the skill or experience to prescribe them safely. When taking Chinese herbs, always follow the dosage advice given by your practitioner.

How acupuncture works

The most widely accepted theory today of how acupuncture works is that it interferes with pain messages to the brain by distracting the brain in a similar way to TENS (see page 83) or by promoting the release of the neurotransmitters called endorphins, which inhibit the transmission of pain (see page 15). The effect may also be due to an increase in ACTH (adrenocorticotropic hormone) from the pituitary gland in the brain. This hormone controls the production of steroid hormones in the kidneys and is used to treat conditions such as asthma and rheumatoid arthritis.

Moxibustion and cupping

Two variations of acupuncture are the techniques known as moxibustion and cupping. In moxibustion a gentle heat is applied to an energy point using moxa, a dried herb (usually common mugwort), because it is believed that this draws and heats the energy, making it more available. The moxa is either attached to the needle so that the heat transfers down it to the energy point or it is rolled into small cones and slowly burned over the point on top of a protective covering.

Cupping uses small cups or jars, often made of glass, to stimulate and draw the body's energy points in much the same way as moxibustion. A lighted taper is held inside the jar and then removed to create a vacuum. The jar clamps itself to the body and sucks on the point. For local inflammation and congestion, cupping is often combined with needles.

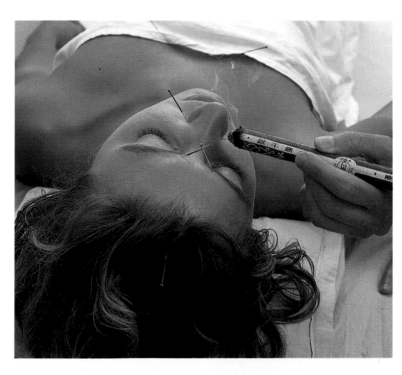

The traditional Oriental concept of meridians means that needles placed on points on the face can relieve symptoms as diverse as sinusitis, stomach complaints, and back pain. Heat may be applied by moxibustion.

Homeopathy

This wide-ranging therapeutic system is based on the recognition that the symptoms of an illness are the body's process of self-healing. Tiny amounts of homeopathic medicines are prescribed. These stimulate the development of the symptoms and thus encourage the body to work through the illness.

A German doctor, Dr. Samuel Hahnemann, developed the system of homeopathic treatment some 200 years ago. He had grown disillusioned with the crude and often brutal medicine of his time and became involved in experiments (often on himself) with medicines and the principles on which they work. He discovered that a very small amount of what causes a disease can also cure it. This gave rise to his principle of "like cures like" and it is the basic principle of homeopathic remedies and treatment.

Homeopathic remedies are made by taking only the smallest amounts of a specific substance, usually from plants or minerals but occasionally also from insects and animals, diluting them in water and/or alcohol and shaking them vigorously, a process known as succussion. This diluting and shaking is done several times. Unlike conventional medicine—in which the greater the concentration of a drug the stronger it is —homeopathy holds that the remedy becomes more potent each time it is diluted and shaken—hence the term "potentization" to describe it. Homeopathic remedies are usually given as small white tablets onto which the potentized mixture has been dripped. Homeopaths, like most natural therapists, see physical symptoms of disease as a manifestation

Homeopathic remedies have no unpleasant side effects and can be used as simple self-help remedies for a number of common conditions.

of deeper problems and will take a detailed history of their patients to try to reveal what is wrong, emotionally and mentally as well as physically, before prescribing. Self-prescribing is useful for simple, common complaints but is not recommended by homeopaths to obtain the best results, even though homeopathic remedies are widely available.

Homeopathy provides no explanation acceptable to scientists on why and how it works but clinical trials appear to show that it does work for some illnesses, and a growing number of doctors now specialize in it. Some studies have shown positive results with animals. Advocates of homeopathy argue that this is significant because, although it is possible that humans respond to what is known as the "placebo effect" (believing their treatment will work and so it does), animals cannot respond in this way. (Detractors say that observers may be biased.)

It is quite common to feel worse after the first homeopathic treatment. This is said to be because the medicine is bringing out the symptoms, but it also appears that homeopathy may work better for some patients than others. Illnesses which are found to respond well to homeopathic treatments include asthma and skin diseases such as eczema.

Most homeopaths insist that general diagnosis is not possible in homeopathy. They also caution that the effectiveness of many homeopathic remedies can be cancelled by other remedies and therapies.

HOMEOPATHIC REMEDIES AND THEIR USES

ACONITE	Shock, illness (especially colds and the flu), coughs, earache, sore throat, stress, toothache
APIS MEL	Stings, cystitis, urethritis, hay fever (allergic rhinitis) and similar allergic reactions, urticaria, arthritis, conjunctivitis
ARNICA	Shock, injury, bruising, sprains, boils, cramps, muscle pain, burns, stings, eye pain, dental pain, fatigue, arthritis, gout, eczema
ARSENICUM ALB	Phlegm, hay fever (allergic rhinitis), diarrhea, food poisoning, vomiting, nausea, fatigue, indigestion, canker sores, urticaria, psoriasis, shingles, insomnia
BELLADONNA	Colds, sore throat, coughs, earaches, headaches, migraines, fever, acne, boils, period pains, sunburn
BRYONIA	Constipation, coughs, colds and the flu, headaches, migraines, indigestion, nausea, arthritis, sore throat, sprains, joint pain, painful breasts
CANTHARIS	Cystitis, nonspecific urethritis, burns, scalds, stings, blisters, canker sores, sunburn, burning diarrhea
CHAMOMILLA	Postdental/surgical pain, teething, insomnia
EUPHRASIA	Colds and the flu, headaches, hay fever (allergic rhinitis), eye pain/strain, conjunctivitis, constipation
GELSEMIUM	Colds and the flu, headaches, migraines, aching joints, sore throat, hay fever (allergic rhinitis), fatigue
HYPERICUM	Crush injuries, cuts and grazes, nerve pain, indigestion, nausea, diarrhea, depression
IGNATIA	Sharp headache, migraine, depression, shock, cough
NATRUM MUR	Grief, depression, colds and the flu, phlegm, cold sores, eczema, hay fever (allergic rhinitis), headache, migraine, PMS, painful periods, urticaria
NUX VOMICA	Constipation, stomachache, colitis, hangover headache, indigestion, sore throat, nausea, motion sickness, vomiting, depression, cystitis, insomnia
PULSATILLA	Sinusitis, colds and the flu, coughs, earache, headache, depression, cystitis, indigestion, stomachache, painful periods, premenstrual syndrome, arthritis, conjunctivitis
RHUS TOX	Blisters, eczema, urticaria, arthritis, sprains, muscle pain, cramps, herpes pain (shingles, cold sores), sore throat
RUTA GRAV	Sprains and strains, sports injuries, muscle pain, arthritic pain, sciatica, headache, eye pain
SILICA	Infected skin, boils, recurring colds, recurring flu, sinusitis, constipation, headache, migraines, fractures
SULFUR	Infected acne, indigestion, constipation, diarrhea, eczema, headache, phlegm, conjunctivitis, joint and muscle pain, cramps, low back pain
URTICA	Burns, scalds, stings, urticaria, cystitis, nerve pain, arthritic pain, allergic skin reactions

Note: These remedies are those most often used for the conditions listed but most homeopaths insist that maximum effectiveness can only be achieved by consultation with an experienced practitioner.

Healing

Many healers believe that they help cure people by transmitting a life force.

M*any people believe that cures can be effected by certain people who have a power to channel a healing power merely by touch or sometimes only by thought. Cases have been attested through the centuries of "faith healing" or "spiritual healing," although healers prefer to simply call it healing because no one really knows how it works.*

Its very simplicity makes healing probably the simplest, safest, and most natural of all methods of therapy and there is more evidence in favor of the therapeutic effects of hands-on healing than any other form of natural therapy, apart from hypnotherapy.

Healing may well be connected in its efficacy with hypnotherapy in that clearly the relationship of healer to patient is all-important. The healer may be a person with special mental or spiritual powers (many religious leaders are credited with faith cures) and the patient usually has to believe in this power for the treatment to be effective.

The treatment does not manipulate the body in any way or involve ingesting medicines of any kind. Patients with any kind of pain may be helped by healing. But, because the personal qualities of the healer are what is supplying the healing, you may have to try several healers before you find one that "works" for you.

Healers vary in their approach to the patient. Some will rely on intuition and touch alone and will "feel" what is wrong with you. Others will ask you questions about your specific problem and your life in general.

Most conventional doctors do not accept the efficacy of this sort of healing. But the interaction of body and mind is still more extensive than we know and, whatever the mechanism, healing has been shown to work for many people and can sometimes achieve dramatic results. Evidence that those people who feel they have been treated positively by their doctor recover better from disease may be part of this same mechanism.

THERAPEUTIC TOUCH

Dolores Krieger, an American professor of nursing, developed therapeutic touch, or "TT," a version of healing using the laying-on-of-hands, in the 1970s.

TT is based on the belief that there is an actual transfer of healing energy from the person touching to the person being touched. It is now in common and increasing use by nurses in clinics and hospitals—particularly in the United States, where to call yourself a healer and to claim to heal by psychic or supernatural means is illegal.

REIKI

Created by a Japanese priest, Dr. Mikao Usui, in the early part of the 20th century, reiki healing has become popular and widespread in recent years. Reiki (pronounced "ray-kee") means "universal life force" in Japanese and is claimed to be the rediscovery of an ancient Tibetan Buddhist technique of healing that involves the transfer of healing energies from one person to the next.

There are now reiki centers in North and South America, Europe, and Australasia as well as Japan, and there are more than 250,000 practitioners worldwide.

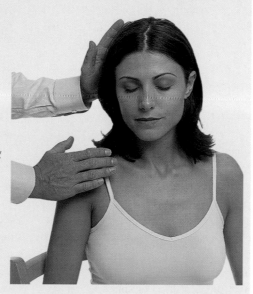

CASE HISTORY

Carol, a shop owner, had healing in 1996 for nerve and eyesight problems that accompanied her multiple sclerosis.

"I was suffering with pains and getting tingling up and down my spine, I had numbness in my legs, and the sight in one eye had become blurred and cloudy. I had been seeing doctors and specialists for about 18 months but all they could come up with after lots of tests was that I had MS and advised me where to get a wheelchair and incontinence pads.

I had been feeling really ill one day when Wendy came into my shop and offered to help. At first I must admit I was very dubious about her, thinking she might be deranged or something, but she said I was not to worry and she would send me absent healing.

I took it with a pinch of salt and felt nothing that day. But the next day I felt much better, and the next day better still. I could hardly believe it. My back and eyesight both improved and the improvements just kept going on. I visited her regularly after that.

The next time I went to see my nerve specialist she could hardly believe it herself. I would be bouncing around like a rubber ball. I still see Wendy for healing, and even though I still have some bad days when my eye plays up and my back hurts, I always feel better after seeing her. The great thing is knowing that she's always there when I need her— and that she always helps."

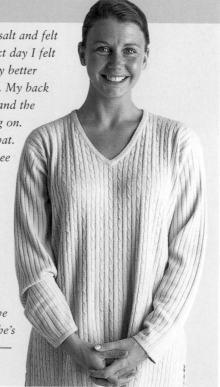

Reflexology

Reflexology is said to be a modern revival of a healing method widely practiced in the ancient world. It can be simply described as foot and hand massage, but most therapists insist it offers much more.

Reflexology has links with acupressure and acupuncture and so is classified as an energy therapy rather than a physical therapy. However, this categorization has been challenged by many reflexologists, who see their work as broadly in line with other physical therapies. This view is held by the Chartered Society of Physiotherapists, the British body for physical therapists, which in 1993 officially recognized reflexology as a physical therapy.

Origins of reflexology

Reflexology is based on the Chinese concept that meridian lines of energy run through the body and link all the major organs to specific reflex points which, in the case of reflexology, are those found in the feet. According to reflexologists, the bottom of each foot can be mapped with areas or zones that correspond to various body organs. By putting the reflex points under pressure, change can be effected in the state of the organs.

A reflexology session

Thumb and finger pressure is applied in much the same way as in acupressure. If no pain is experienced the organ is deemed to be sound, but any discomfort is said to indicate a problem in the

A reflexology treatment should be a relaxing experience, with both therapist and patient sitting comfortably.

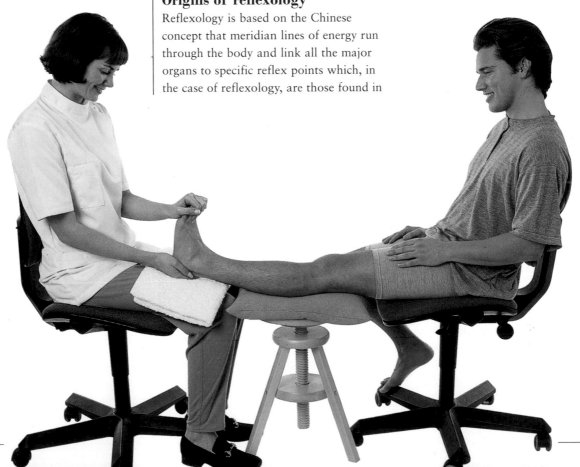

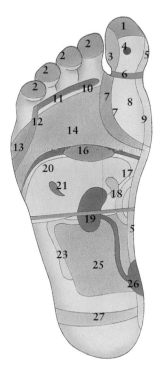

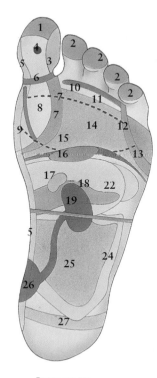

RIGHT FOOT   LEFT FOOT

Find out more

What to expect from
a therapist   28
Acupressure   38

REFLEXOLOGY POINTS ON THE FEET

1 Brain	15 Heart
2 Sinuses	16 Solar plexus
3 Side of neck	17 Stomach
4 Pituitary gland	18 Pancreas
5 Spine	19 Kidney
6 Neck	20 Liver
7 Parathyroid	21 Gallbladder
8 Thyroid	22 Spleen
9 Trachea	23 Ascending colon
10 Eyes	24 Descending colon
11 Eustachian tube	25 Small intestine
12 Ear	26 Bladder
13 Shoulder	27 Sciatic nerve
14 Lung	

corresponding area of the body, so further pressure is applied. This may be distinctly uncomfortable, but therapists say that by working on the point for a few moments the pain usually eases and a response is felt in the affected organ. For example, a headache might be relieved by having pressure applied to the base of the big toe, which in reflexology corresponds to the base of the neck, and chest congestion can be cleared by pressing the ball of the foot, corresponding to the lungs.

Reflexology does not claim to be able to remove inflammation or infection, but therapists do claim that treatment can speed up and help maintain recovery. Most patients say the therapy is relaxing and the massage helps improve circulation and benefits most bodily functions,

whether it helps individual organs or not. Many people say they feel like resting or sleeping after a treatment, which is possibly due to the release of enkephalin and endorphin hormones.

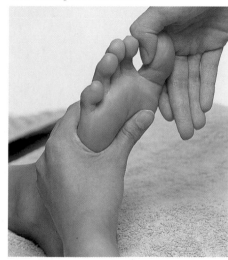

In reflexology the base of the big toe corresponds to the base of the neck and the ball of the foot to the lungs. Massaging and pressing these areas eases neck and lung pain.

CHAPTER TWO

Psychotherapy treatments

*T**alking** about yourself and your problems to a trained and experienced listener can often help you understand the causes of mental or emotional pain and express feelings which you may have buried. Psychotherapists and counselors work with their clients to move toward finding solutions.*

Mental or emotional pain can be buried in us from childhood or it can be the result of some recent trauma, such as bereavement or a problem in a relationship. Psychotherapy and counseling give the client the freedom to explore and express emotions and thoughts that they previously have not wished to voice or confront, in absolute confidentiality. In most Western countries it is becoming increasingly common to find professional counselors and psychotherapists allied to doctors' offices, health centers, and clinics.

Counseling

Counseling can be an extremely effective way of helping many people cope with periods of major emotional stress and strain, caused perhaps by a failed relationship, being laid off at

work, or sexual problems. Many counselors specialize in one of these areas and will see you on a one-to-one basis or perhaps with a partner or other family members.

Psychotherapy

As with counseling, psychotherapy is a method of allowing people to talk through emotional and mental problems and receive support and guidance for them. However, psychotherapy also goes much further, tackling the deeper, often hidden, underlying causes of emotional distress by trying to get the client to understand and face up to psychological problems within themselves. This can be done on either an individual basis or as part of a group.

Psychotherapy developed out of psychoanalysis when both clients and practitioners began to be critical of the more analytical approach of the science pioneered by Sigmund Freud. There are now many types and styles of approach, from the complex (psychoanalysis) to the down-to-earth (laughter therapy), each suited to different people and problems.

Some psychotherapists will mostly sit and listen to you, others will work more actively through creating situations (simulating work or relationships), by encouraging the release of childhood

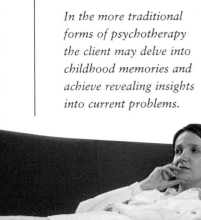

In the more traditional forms of psychotherapy the client may delve into childhood memories and achieve revealing insights into current problems.

emotions, or by following a course of gradual desensitization for a phobia.

Therapists—and this includes a growing numbers of doctors—who specialize in any of these approaches tend to be familiar with the other types and will guide someone to the right analyst if they cannot help that person themselves.

Hypnotherapy

A variety of problems can be helped by hypnotherapy. Some psychological problems can be quite specific, such as addictions or fears; others may go back to some trauma, which the patient cannot consciously remember. Disorders which may have a psychosomatic cause, such as skin complaints or an irritable bowel, can also be helped by hypnotherapy.

This is achieved by the hypnotherapist inducing a state of deep relaxation in the client. The nature of this is not fully understood, but before anesthetics were discovered, some surgeons induced a state of trance in patients in order to operate on them painlessly, so the power of the suggestion lies very deep and is very effective. The patient is enabled to get in touch with the deep-rooted cause of their problem or to imagine ways in which they could cope more easily. Once the cause is known—it may be a specific event such as a childhood trauma or it may be more general, such as deeply rooted guilt about something—the client may be advised to deal with it consciously by undergoing standard counseling or psychotherapy. This is why some hypnotherapists are also trained psychotherapists.

Hypnotherapy is also a way of learning to relax on a deep level. The many tapes now available use a form of hypnosis to aid relaxation, although some therapists do not recommend them.

WARNING

It is not possible to force someone to perform an act against his or her will when in a trance. However, it is important to check the credentials of your therapist thoroughly before agreeing to treatment. Ask your doctor for a referral or check that the practitioner is registered with a recognized professional organization and ask for its details.

Find out more

Self-hypnosis	46
Emotional pain	90

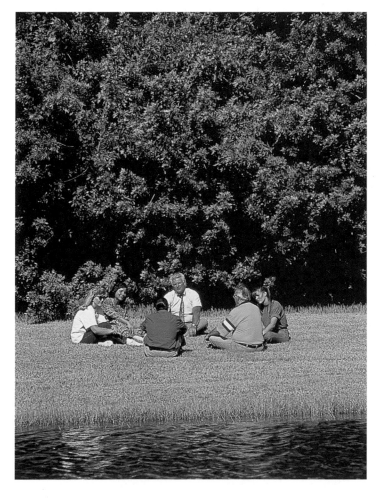

Many people find that talking with others in a group setting can alleviate anxiety and distress.

Medical specialists

Y*our doctor may refer you to a specialist if your treatments have not worked, or further investigations are needed after blood tests and X rays have been carried out, or if your symptoms do not fit any recognizable pattern.*

In the chart below, M indicates a medical qualification, D a dental qualification.

A specialist, or consultant, is a highly trained and experienced doctor with an in-depth knowledge of your type of problem. A specialist will check your medical history, take a case history, and examine you. Further X rays might be carried out or, if they do not give enough information, a scan may be required.

SPECIALISTS AND THEIR AREAS OF EXPERTISE	
AUDIOLOGISTS	Concerned with hearing disorders, audiologists diagnose hearing problems. They work in tandem with ear, nose, and throat specialists.
CARDIOLOGISTS (M)	Doctors who specialize in heart problems, cardiologists are concerned with the diagnosis and management of heart conditions. They do not perform surgery.
DERMATOLOGISTS (M)	Dermatologists diagnose and treat a wide range of skin problems.
DIETITIANS AND NUTRITIONISTS	Many problems can arise—and cause pain—by following an inadequate diet. People with digestive, metabolic, and malnutritional disorders are frequently referred to dietitians and nutritionists.
ENDOCRINOLOGISTS (M)	These are specialists who deal with problems of the endocrine system, which releases hormones into the bloodstream.
GASTROENTEROLOGISTS (M)	These are doctors specializing in the disorders of the digestive system and their associated glands, such as the liver and pancreas.
GENITO-URINARY SPECIALISTS (M)	These specialists are concerned with urinary problems, as well as the physical consequences of sexually transmitted diseases.
GERIATRICIANS (M)	These are doctors specializing in the care and treatment of old people. Pain management may be included in their job.
GYNECOLOGISTS (M)	Disorders of the female reproductive system—many of which cause severe pain— are diagnosed and treated by these doctors.

There are many specialized tests that can be done to find the cause of your problem. The specialist will then discuss your options for treatment with you and will tell your doctor so that you can talk with him or her too.

You should remember that you have the right to know everything about your treatment and can refuse any part of it which you do not want.

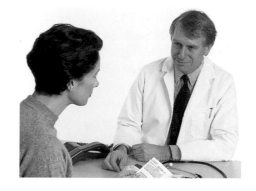

Find out more

SPECIALISTS AND THEIR AREAS OF EXPERTISE

NEUROLOGISTS (M)	Problems of the nervous system, including the brain, are diagnosed and treated by neurologists.
ONCOLOGISTS (M)	Oncology is the study of cancer. Oncologists are specialists in the treatment and management of cancer.
ORTHODONTISTS (D)	Orthodontists can help a great deal if the cause of your pain is your "bite," the way your jaw joint is working. An indication of this is if your problems include head, neck, or shoulder pains.
ORTHOPEDISTS (M)	These specialists diagnose and treat problems to do with the skeletal system and everything that makes it move.
ORTHOTISTS	Orthotics is the service that provides custom-made mechanical aids, such as corsets, limbs, shoe-lifts, and other appliances.
PAIN SPECIALISTS (M)	Doctors drawn from one or more specialities who offer a multidisciplinary approach to pain relief
PODIATRISTS	Podiatrists treat diseases, injuries, and abnormalities of the foot.
PSYCHOLOGISTS AND psychiatrists (M)	These specialists diagnose and treat problems of the mind that may either be the cause of the pain or a result of it. (Note: Psychologists are not MDs.)
RHEUMATOLOGISTS (M)	Rheumatologists diagnose and treat people with inflammatory disorders, such as rheumatoid arthritis and ankylosing spondylitis.
SURGEONS (M)	Surgeons specialize in internal manipulation or operation; subspecialities include genitourinary, general, gynecological, and orthopedic surgery.

Drug therapy

Drugs for pain comprise those you can buy over the counter in your local pharmacy (self-help) and those that only a doctor can prescribe for you. Over-the-counter drugs are generally weaker and so less potentially dangerous than those prescribed by your doctor.

MAIN CLASSES OF DRUGS FOR PAIN	
PAINKILLERS (ANALGESICS)	Analgesics "kill" pain by reducing the pain response in the brain. They include such widely used drugs as aspirin and the morphinelike drugs, of which codeine is a weak synthetic version. Though many are commonly available over the counter in most countries, they are not without side effects and are dangerous in excess.
NONSTEROIDAL ANTI-INFLAMMATORIES (NSAIDs)	These drugs have anti-inflammatory effects, and also analgesic effects, and include aspirin, ibuprofen, diclofenac, indomethacin, mefenamic acid, naproxen, and piroxicam. They may cause ulcers and seriously exacerbate asthma. Part of their analgesic effect is as a result of their anti-inflammatory action. Creams or gels are available and can be as effective as tablets.
MUSCLE RELAXANTS	These are tranquillizers that have a relaxing effect on the muscles. Similar doses are used to relax muscle spasms as for treating anxiety. This range of drugs is very addictive and so they are usually prescribed for short-term use. One of the best known examples is diazepam. Tranquillizers work as a brain sedative, even at low doses, and so can cause loss of concentration and poor memory.
ANTIDEPRESSANTS	Tricyclic antidepressants (amitriptyline, imipramine, desipramine) given in small doses—insufficient to have an effect on depression—can be as effective as analgesics. They cause sedation and are therefore given at night, and may help sleep and also a dry mouth. Like all drugs that affect the brain, they may have unwelcome side effects.
STEROIDS	These are also anti-inflammatory drugs and are effective in relieving pain due to inflammation, and also to reduce swelling where nerves are being compressed. They also have a long-lasting local anesthetic effect when injected. They can cause stomach ulcers, Cushing's syndrome (a serious hormonal disease), and osteoporosis.

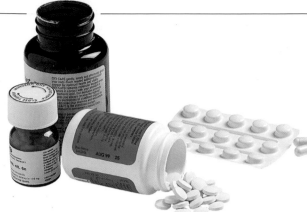

Drug therapy is one of the basic treatments provided by conventional medicine. Many find such drugs produce side effects.

INJECTION TREATMENTS

FACET JOINT INJECTIONS	These usually contain a steroid and an anesthetic. They can give relief lasting from just a few hours to about a month (in up to 15 percent of cases), as is the case with severe arthritis. These are best used as an aid to diagnosis to ascertain whether facet joint denervation is appropriate.
STEROID INJECTIONS	These are injected into the facet joints (see above), other inflamed joints, sprained ligaments, and muscles. They are sometimes combined with cooling spray and stretching exercises if there are "trigger points" within the muscle **WARNING**: Repeated steroid injections cause weakening of the bones, ligaments, and muscle attachments around the site of the injections.
SCLEROSANT INJECTIONS	These are injections to "sclerose" or harden and tighten ligaments that have become too lax and floppy. The injections contain an irritant solution that causes extra fibrous tissue to form around the site of injection. Injections are carried out weekly and each injection lasts about 15 minutes. Although injections can be given under a mild anesthetic, they are painful and the full effects are not apparent for a couple of months. There is no guarantee of long-term benefit but some people have been pain-free for years after treatment. This may be due in part to the fact that they destroy nerves in the vicinity of the injection.
EPIDURAL INJECTIONS	Injections of anesthetics and steroids into the spinal canal are given to numb pain due to compression of a nerve, usually by a disk protrusion. The steroid may reduce the swelling around the disk, reducing pressure on the nerve. The injection allows you to "play for time" and let the body break down the damaged disk by itself, with the aim of overcoming the need for other treatments. However, if nerve damage leads to motor weakness or urinary problems, surgery may be necessary. Most disk problems are not protrusions and heal in their own time.
CHEMONUCLEOLYSIS	An enzyme made from the papaya fruit is injected into the soft nucleus of protruding disks to dissolve them. It will shrink a bulging disk permanently but it can also cause severe disk collapse, putting more pressure on surrounding joints. It is not used for severe protrusions with floating disk particles around them. Sometimes the drug can leak into sensitive surrounding areas, causing soreness.

Physiotherapy

A variety of musculoskeletal problems can be helped by physiotherapy, which is normally the only manual ("hands-on") therapy offered by conventional medicine. Your initial appointment will be similar to one with your family doctor.

A physiotherapist will give you a thorough examination before deciding on the most appropriate treatment for you.

Your doctor may recommend physiotherapy for recovery from breaks and sprains, or more persistent pain in the back or joints. Most hospitals have a physiotherapy department, and physiotherapists also often work in health centers. They can offer a variety of treatments and many train in specialist areas as well. They will usually monitor your progress over a series of visits.

Manipulation

Physiotherapy treatment usually involves joint articulation and manipulation. Articulation is moving joints in a controlled way to diagnose problems or to increase the range of movement around a joint.

Physiotherapists use the so-called Maitlands mobilization technique, which uses a graded series of hand pressures to stretch and move joints within a comfortable range. This eases the "bind" of tight muscles, adhesions, scarred joint capsules, and so on, and it also improves the exchange of body fluids in and out of the joints.

Massage

Physiotherapists also use massages and exercises, sharing the philosophy of many complementary manipulative therapists that the body will correct itself if the right exercises are given. The range of exercises is wide and many are almost identical to those used in yoga.

Hydrotherapy

Water therapy, or hydrotherapy, has also been used by physiotherapists for many years and its therapeutic qualities in treating pain are widely recognized.

Hydrotherapy usually involves being guided through a series of controlled movements by the therapist in a large pool of warm water (swimming pools are often used). The physiotherapist is usually in the pool with you to guide your movements and correct your posture.

Unlike naturopathic hydrotherapy, which uses a variety of sometimes quite involved techniques, hydrotherapy in physiotherapy is used simply to take advantage of the buoyancy of water. Because the water supports much of a person's body weight, thus taking pressure off painful joints and muscles, it makes it easier to exercise. It also means that a person is less likely to suffer an exercise-related injury.

Traction

Physiotherapists also use traction, which literally means "pulling." It is carried out manually or with sometimes quite elaborate, even uncomfortable-looking, machines into which the sufferer is strapped. Used mainly to help with back problems, the aim of traction is to stretch tissues to take pressure off disks. Mechanical traction is also used in hospitals for people in extreme pain from nerve-root pressure, but it is both unpopular (patients are strapped in for long periods and not usually allowed toilet breaks) and controversial. Some pain experts contend that the enforced bed rest involved with traction causes more problems than it solves, including constipation, and that it has no real long-term benefit. Nevertheless, it is clear that it does help some people.

The use of electronic pain-relieving devices also has a valuable role to play in pain relief (see box below).

ELECTRONIC PAIN-RELIEVING DEVICES

TENS

TENS (transcutaneous electrical nerve stimulation) uses a device that sends electrical impulses from a battery to the nerves via electrodes attached to the surface of the skin, usually on or near the site of the ache or pain or over the nerves supplying that area. It works on the principle of the gate control theory. One theory holds that it makes certain cells in the spinal cord less responsive to pain signals, blocking their transmission to the brain; another that the electrical impulses stimulate the production of endorphins to block the perception of pain.

TENS is a useful therapy for certain types of pain, providing relief for 30 to 50 percent of sufferers of chronic pain. Recent developments mean that TENS devices are now available for home use. They are also usually available for rent.

A more sophisticated version is Giga-TENS. This claims to achieve much more dramatic results by pulsing just a billionth of a watt at 52–78 GHz (billion cycles per second). Described as "solar acupuncture" by the pioneering American neurosurgeon Dr Norman Shealy (who claims it is potentially the most powerful healing tool ever discovered), Giga-TENS remains controversial and so is unlikely to be widely available for many years.

INTERFERENTIAL THERAPY

Small levels of opposing electrical currents are set up to "interfere" with each other. Applied to areas of pain by suckers or moist sponges, the therapy produces a tingling sensation that can give short-term pain relief.

SHORT-WAVE DIATHERMY

Also known as pulsed electromagnetic energy (PEME), this uses pulsed electromagnetic waves to speed up healing. It is effective on fractures that are slow to heal and for treating soft-tissue damage.

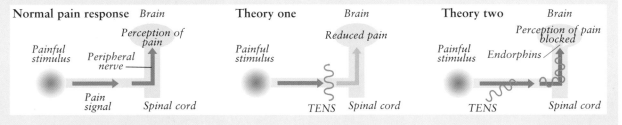

Normal pain response — Brain, Perception of pain, Painful stimulus, Peripheral nerve, Pain signal, Spinal cord

Theory one — Brain, Reduced pain, Painful stimulus, TENS, Spinal cord

Theory two — Brain, Perception of pain blocked, Painful stimulus, Endorphins, TENS, Spinal cord

Medical imaging tests

Conventional medicine can offer a variety of ways of producing images of your problem in order to diagnose it. This is most likely to happen if your pain is severe, prolonged, or recurrent. Medical imaging requires expensive equipment and so has to be done at a hospital or large medical center.

Diagnostic tests range from blood tests and X rays to the more sophisticated scanning techniques. There is a wide range of blood tests available but their purpose is the same: to analyze the chemical content of blood to check for signs of irregularities and disease.

X rays

A picture can be taken using ultra short-wave radiation called X rays. The X rays are absorbed by the bones and some other body tissues, which show up dark on the print. The pictures can provide information about bones and teeth and identify stones and cancers. Because of the radiation, however, X rays should be used sparingly.

CT (CAT) scan

Computerized tomography (CT) uses very small quantities of X rays (one second for

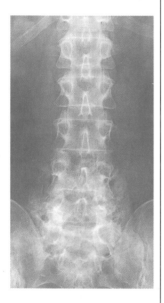

X rays are still useful, giving an overview of the bone structure, but more sophisticated imaging techniques can show other tissues to give a picture of the nerves and soft tissues. X rays are also inexpensive, while scans are still costly.

the whole head) linked to a revolving scanning device that records the different thicknesses of tissues and translates them onto film for analysis. Unlike X rays, which penetrate the whole body and so give a general and sometimes not very clear view, a CT scan is very specific, producing a highly accurate picture of even a very thin layer of tissue.

Ultrasound scan

This is a quick and painless method of looking deep into the body. It works by picking up the amount of "echo" produced by different solid human tissues and converting their sound waves into an image that can be analyzed. Like CT scans, ultrasound is a useful diagnostic tool for use on tissues where exploratory surgery would be a high-risk procedure, but it is of no use in the brain where the skull bones obscure the tissue.

MAGNETIC RESONANCE IMAGING SCAN

Magnetic resonance imaging (MRI) works in a similar way to a CT scan but uses extremely powerful electromagnets and radio waves instead of X rays. It is one of the best tests for nerve damage, examination of joints, soft tissue, and the detection of disorders of and injuries to the spine.

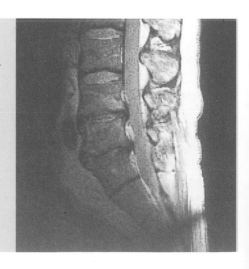

Myelogram

The myelogram test (also called radiculography) is normally only used when surgery is being considered on the spine for severe musculoskeletal problems. A dye is injected into the spinal canal and allowed to spread around the nerve roots and spinal cord. This then shows up on an X ray film and enables the surgeon to identify which nerves are affected. The dyes used, particularly the older, oil-based ones, have a mixed safety record.

Electromyography

In electromyography, fine needles are inserted into the muscles to measure their electrical activity. For example, if the problem is back pain due to suspected disk disease, the muscles in the leg, calf, or foot will be tested because they are the muscles most commonly affected by disk disease. If the response of a muscle group is weak, this indicates that the nerve roots in the spine between the spinal cord and the muscles are a problem.

Endoscopy

This is a technique of viewing the internal organs by means of a long, thin, flexible viewing tube. The surgeon views the organs either directly through a lens or relayed on to a monitor.

Electrocardiogram (EKG)

An EKG measures the rhythm and electrical activity of the heart to identify abnormalities such as heart disease. It is usually done under "resting" conditions, but between 25 and 50 percent of all resting tests can give a "false negative" result, showing no abnormalities when there is heart disease; or a "false positive" result, where an abnormal reading is

shown despite there being no heart problem. A high degree of skill and experience is therefore essential in interpreting results.

Computer image fusion

This is a new, computerized imaging and navigational aid that produces a static picture and allows surgeons to go directly to the affected area with great accuracy. It is suitable for the diagnosis and treatment of spinal problems, including the removal of diseased disks or tumors.

As a patient lies within the rotating detector of a CT scanner, an image of a section of her brain is displayed on a viewing screen.

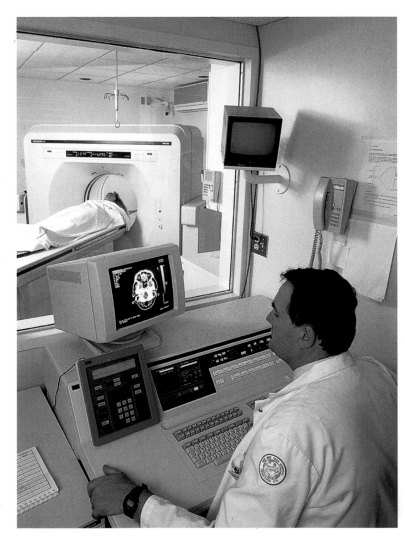

Surgery

*I*f your pain is caused by an organ that is malfunctioning or by damage from an accident, you may have to undergo surgery as the only recourse. Many operations are now routine and microsurgery techniques minimize trauma.

There are different types of surgeons you are likely to be referred to if your doctor thinks surgery is necessary.

Neurosurgeons operate on the skull and spinal column and their contents (so they will handle, for example, operations for brain injury or disease, or a slipped or damaged disk in the spine). Orthopedic surgeons do more "repositioning" work, for example, on fractures, deformities, joint replacements, and soft tissues. A gastro-intestinal surgeon would remove stones from the digestive tract.

Modern technology has meant that the safety and sophistication of operations has increased rapidly in recent years and many operations are now done "blind"

through tiny cuts in the skin using a binocular microscope and continuous imaging to guide the surgical instruments. (see box on keyhole surgery, right).

However, the patient will rarely be pain-free immediately after an operation so a commitment to sustained work is usually necessary to regain full function of the affected area if the problem has been a long-standing one.

Weighing the risks

Surgery is usually regarded as a last resort as a cure for pain of most kinds—especially back pain—because the results are variable and it is still the most invasive treatment option. There are risks

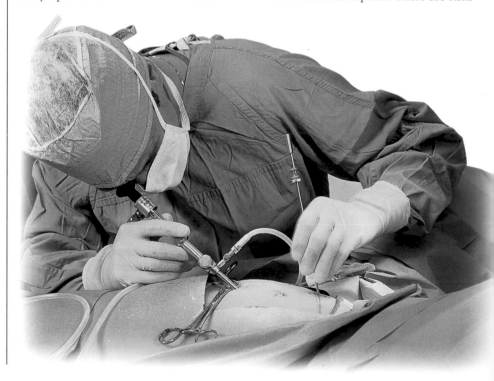

A surgeon views the interior of the body with an endoscope and so avoids having to make a large incision to perform an operation.

involved in any operation, such as a reaction to the anesthetic, chest infection, blood clots, infection of the wound, and hemorrhage (sudden and severe blood loss, very occasionally needing a blood transfusion). In the case of spinal surgery, there are particular risks such as spinal nerve or spinal cord damage, which can lead in rare cases to some form of paralysis. This occurs in one out of every 5,000 operations.

Statistically, the death rate from operations is low. For example, there is approximately a 1 in 300 chance of death during or as a result of a spinal operation —which is usually the result of severe damage to the spinal cord or from a blood clot in the lungs.

Fears about an operation should be talked through with your doctor and surgeon and you should not be pressured into going ahead until you feel satisfied that the potential benefits significantly outweigh the risks. Good doctors will back you in a cautious approach.

Find out more

Physiotherapy   82
Medical imaging tests 84

KEYHOLE SURGERY

A relatively recent development, keyhole surgery is also known as minimally invasive surgery. Only tiny incisions need to be made— much smaller than in conventional surgery. This means that the procedure avoids leaving a long scar and recovery after an operation is very quick: You might be able to go home within two or three days and may find that there is almost no visible scarring at all.

The surgeon uses a viewing device called an endoscope. In some procedures, the endoscope is fitted with a miniature video camera that transmits an image onto a screen. Otherwise the surgeon looks directly through an eyepiece.

The endoscope also carries a range of surgical attachments such as forceps and a scalpel within flexible tubing.

The surgeon makes incisions of about 1/2 inch (10 millimeters) in diameter for the camera or viewing device and the other instruments and, viewing through the endoscope, manipulates them to the precise area to be operated on.

Sometimes the procedure uses lasers instead of scalpels to cut tissues and many other standard surgical instruments have been specially adapted and miniaturized for use in keyhole surgery.

Endoscopes have different names depending on the region of the body where they are used—for example, an arthroscope is used for the joints and a laparoscope is used for the stomach cavity.

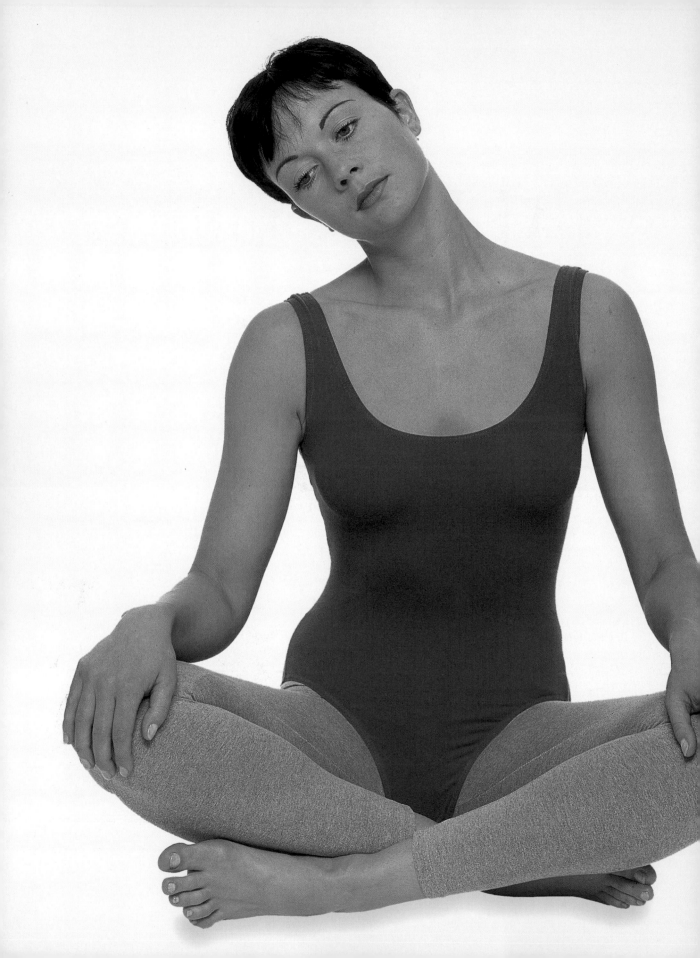

3

ALLEVIATING

PAIN

There are many ways of alleviating pain, from conventional medicine to complementary therapies. This chapter looks at some of the most common causes of pain divided according to general areas of the body and including nerve, joint, and muscle pain, circulatory pain, skin pain, and psychological pain, among others. The focus here is on complementary therapies, such as herbal medicine, massage, dietary and nutritional therapies, yoga, t'ai chi, and naturopathy. Although some alternative treatments, such as acupuncture, should be applied only by a qualified practitioner, most can be administered either by the patient after an introductory session with an alternative therapist, such as a homeopath, or be self-administered, for example, aromatherapy.

Treatments for emotional pain

*T*he concept that pain is emotional as well as physical is an unfamiliar one to many—except those who experience it. Emotional trauma can produce depression and anxiety and, in severe cases, can lead to physical pain.

Psychological distress as a result of emotional trauma, such as grief over the loss of a loved one, or feelings of rejection, can lead to depression. In extreme cases this may lead to physical pain since the areas of the brain that deal with emotional suffering are the same as those that deal with physical pain.

Nutritional and dietary therapies
Vitamin and mineral deficiencies may exacerbate some types of depression because chemical imbalances in the body can affect hormone levels—and hormones play a major part in mood. Finding out if this is a factor calls for the help of a specialist who will need to carry out

HOW DEPRESSED ARE YOU?

If you know you are experiencing emotional pain or distress but do not know why or how badly, try the self-assessment questionnaire below. Evidence shows that the more people know about the causes of their mental and emotional pain or depression, the more likely they are to overcome it successfully. This self-assessment questionnaire, devised by a doctor, will help you assess your frame of mind. If you find you are depressed, you can start to do something effective about it. Rank the following 10 categories from 0 to 4 using your own assessment of how severe each emotion is for you.

	NONE	MILD	MODERATE	SEVERE	VERY SEVERE
DEPRESSED MOOD	0	1	2	3	4
FEELINGS OF GUILT	0	1	2	3	4
SUICIDAL FEELINGS	0	1	2	3	4
CONCENTRATION AND MEMORY PROBLEMS	0	1	2	3	4
FEELINGS OF LASSITUDE	0	1	2	3	4
DISTURBED SLEEP	0	1	2	3	4
LOSS OF SEXUAL DESIRE	0	1	2	3	4
LOSS OF APPETITE	0	1	2	3	4
FEELINGS OF ANXIETY	0	1	2	3	4
SYMPTOMS OF ANXIETY	0	1	2	3	4

After ranking each category, add the scores together to give a total (maximum 40). A score of 10 or under classes you as "normal": You are experiencing what most people feel most of the time. To be classed as depressed you must score at least 2 in the first category, "Depressed mood." The higher the total above 10, the more you should consider trying the treatments on pages 90–95. A score over 30 means you should consult a doctor or other specialist in treating depression.

careful tests. Eating a healthy diet and taking a good multivitamin food supplement containing a broad spectrum of nutrients can be beneficial. The supplement should include vitamins A, B-complex, C, and E; the minerals zinc, calcium, selenium, magnesium, and potassium; and a complex of amino acids.

Herbal medicine

Hypericum (St. John's wort), valerian, rosemary, lavender, and lemon balm are said to be effective against depression, particularly mild depression from tension, anxiety, and insomnia. Hypericum is now widely available since research has proved its effectiveness—but it is necessary to take the recommended dose regularly for up to a month for best results.

Visualization

The power of the mind can be utilized to help the physical body through positive visualization. It can be used by focusing on the distress you are feeling and changing it to relieve depression. Use your image until your mind is in control of the pain, and not the other way around.

Think of a positive image that also contains a solution. Visualize it regularly. Ideally, you will find that your mind will think the pain away.

Creative arts therapies

This therapy encourages emotional expression in a nonverbal way. Many who are unable to find relief through talking, perhaps because they are self-conscious, find this therapy very helpful. ▶

Find out more

Visualization	*50*
Creative arts therapies	*54*
Herbal medicine	*60*

TREATMENT APPROACHES TO EMOTIONAL PAIN

Effective therapies for emotional pain include both physical and psychological approaches, as well as some of the so-called energy therapies. Self-help is possible if the cause of the pain is obvious and the sufferer is confident or willing to treat him- or herself. Knowing or suspecting what is behind the pain is important because if the cause is unknown, effective treatment is difficult, if not impossible.

The help of others is necessary if the cause of the pain is unidentifiable, if it is so severe the sufferer is unable, for several reasons, or unwilling to try self-help, or if special guidance is necessary for the treatment to be effective. Therapies with the best record for helping to ease emotional pain are listed below.

SELF-HELP	**Physical:** Exercise, massage, aromatherapy, reflexology **Psychological:** Meditation, visualization, self-hypnosis, biofeedback **Energy therapies:** Bach flower remedies
SELF-HELP WITH GUIDANCE	**Physical:** Nutrition and dietary therapies, herbal medicine, movement therapies (yoga, t'ai chi, Alexander technique), light and color therapies, flotation therapy **Psychological:** Creative arts therapies (music, art, dance, drama) **Energy therapies:** Homeopathy
PRACTITIONER TREATMENT	**Physical:** Cranial osteopathy **Psychological:** Counseling, psychotherapy, hypnotherapy/hypnosis **Energy therapies:** Acupuncture

Treatments for emotional pain

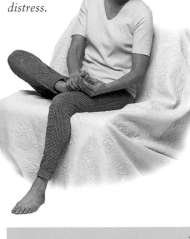

Foot massage is an ideal way to relieve the tension that may be contributing to mental distress.

Meditation

Not only can meditation help calm a mind in turmoil but it can also allow the person meditating to see the world in a wider, less personal way (see pp. 48–49).

When experiencing mental anguish it is easy to believe that you have been singled out for bad luck. During meditation, students are taught to focus outside themselves, which can be a great relief for those who internalize their feelings or find that they are unable to stop fretting about their emotional problems.

Healing

The application of a healing force from outside yourself requires the services of a "healer" to be effective.

Finding someone with this gift for helping people is easier in some countries than others (see pp. 72–73). Personal recommendation is usually the best way to find a genuine healer, as there is no regulatory body.

Exercise

Any form of exercise—especially if it is energetic and distracting—can help with most types of mental and emotional pain. Running, walking, climbing, swimming and cycling are all excellent ways of using exercise to help with psychological pain because they prevent the mind and emotions from taking control. Also, as well as promoting the optimal functioning of the heart and lungs which is essential for health, physical exercise triggers the release of endorphins, the so-called pleasure hormones, which reduce psychological and physical pain. Exercising at the first sign of the onset of mild depression can often stop it in its

ESSENTIAL OILS FOR DEPRESSION

CONDITION OR EFFECT	ESSENTIAL OILS
ANTI-DEPRESSANT AND SEDATIVE	Sandalwood, ylang ylang
MILD DEPRESSION, FEELING "UNDER THE WEATHER"	Lavender, clary sage
DEPRESSION WITH RESTLESSNESS AND IRRITABILITY	Chamomile, clary sage, lavender
DEPRESSION WITH LACK OF CONFIDENCE, FEAR	Jasmine, frankincense, rose
DEPRESSION WITH ANXIETY, INSOMNIA	Neroli, geranium, lavender, rose, vetiver
EMOTIONAL PAIN WITH ANGER	Chamomile, ylang ylang, patchouli
DEEP EMOTIONAL PAIN	Neroli, rose
TO LIFT MOOD WITHOUT SEDATING	Bergamot, geranium, melissa, rose
GENERAL ANTI-DEPRESSANT	Bergamot, frankincense

Warning: Essential oils can be toxic and even lethal if taken internally. Some aromatherapy oils are not suitable for use during pregnancy. Check with your practitioner.

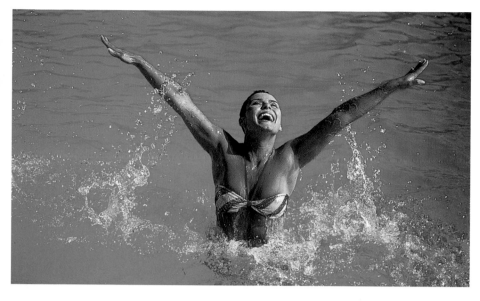

Find out more

Aromatherapy	36
Yoga	40
Reflexology	74

Swimming and aquarobics are excellent forms of exercise, since your body is supported in water and unlikely to suffer any strains. Exercise can promote feelings of well-being that last long after your session is over.

tracks—and it helps strengthen the body against other illnesses that depression can trigger or aggravate.

Aromatherapy

Almost all essential oils used in aromatherapy have a useful role in treating psychological pain, whether they are used for massage or vaporized with a burner and inhaled. The range is large but the oils most favored are shown in the chart (left). Ask for recommendations at a store that supplies them (they are widely available and some stores have samplers for you to try before you buy). Alternatively, seek the advice of a qualified clinical aromatherapist. For massage, mix 2 or 3 drops of the chosen oil(s) in about 2 tsp of a neutral carrier oil such as grapeseed or sweet almond.

Massage

Like exercise, massaging—preferably, being massaged—is a wonderful de-stressor and psychological pain reliever, especially if used with essential oils. There are recognized techniques of massage,

which professional therapists have to learn (see pp. 56–57), but it is possible to improvise for a home massage. Using firm, flowing strokes and doing what you or your partner likes can be relaxing and distract from emotional pain.

Reflexology

Manipulating the soles and sides of the feet is another excellent relaxer that benefits the mind and emotions as much as the body. Reflexology is based on the principle that energy from the entire body flows to the feet. Different parts of the feet relate to different body parts and organs—sections of the big toe correspond to the head and brain. Apply firm pressure with bent thumbs and linger on areas that are tender until the tenderness subsides. For best results consult a professional reflexologist.

Bodywork therapies

Techniques, such as Rolfing, Hellerwork, and the Trager approach can all help, but they need to be administered by a qualified practitioner (see pp. 66–67). ▶

Treatments for emotional pain

Color therapists believe that as light is absorbed it alters the body's chemical balance. By bathing the body in colored light, a therapist can rebalance physical and emotional disturbances.

Movement therapies

The Oriental techniques of yoga and t'ai chi, which combine physical movement with correct breathing and mental concentration, offer profound benefits for those with mental and emotional problems. The range of movements is enormous (a few of the best known are shown on pp. 42–45), so it is best to seek guidance from an experienced practitioner at first. More recently, the Alexander technique, developed in the West, concentrates on improving posture, which can help you feel better about yourself.

Light and color therapies

Light and color are both known to have an effect on our mental, emotional, and physical states. Sunlight deprivation affects the levels of melatonin and serotonin, the "mood" hormones, and causes the depressive winter syndrome known as seasonal affective disorder (SAD). Treatment for SAD involves investing in lighting for the home that mimics natural daylight, known as full-spectrum lighting (FSL), or visiting a center that offers FSL therapeutic treatment. Other research has shown that blue colors are cooling, pinks calming, greens balancing, and reds heating or exciting. You can try this yourself by simply wearing a color you would like to "feel"—blue to calm you, for example, or green to make you more emotionally balanced. If you want to surround yourself with colors likely to be of benefit to you it is best to seek advice from a trained color therapist.

Homeopathy

There are hundreds of homeopathic remedies for every possible type of psychological pain, many of which are linked to physical pain. The need for individual assessment is so vital that it is best to see a professional (see pp. 70–71).

Self-help becomes more appropriate once the right remedy pattern has been established by a specialist. However, you may like to try some of the products available widely from pharmacies to treat temporary, minor emotional upsets.

Bach flower remedies

The British physician Dr. Edward Bach, working at the beginning of the 20th century, believed that the causes of illness were negative emotional states, such as sorrow and fear. He discovered 38 flower remedies, which help relieve feelings such as anxiety, grief, and irritation.

Dr. Bach's remedies can be taken without professional advice. They are made from flower extracts, very dilute, and taken a couple of drops at a time. Each remedy represents an emotional state and you can combine up to six or seven. To select a remedy, think of the type of person you are, as described in the chart (right). For example, if you lack confidence, choose larch. Then look at how you feel now. If, for example, you have just moved to a new town and are feeling unsettled, you could add honeysuckle and walnut. Do not worry if you make the wrong choice—if a remedy is not needed it will have no effect.

THE BACH FLOWER REMEDIES

FLOWER	EMOTIONAL CHARACTERISTICS	FLOWER	EMOTIONAL CHARACTERISTICS
AGRIMONY	Hides anxiety, restless, avoids arguments	MIMULUS	Fear of physical things, timidity, nervousness
ASPEN	Unexplained apprehension, fear from dreams, tired, and nervous	MUSTARD	Intense depression from unknown cause, periodic affliction
BEECH	Critical, dissatisfied, intolerant, always finding fault	OAK	Persevering, obstinate, strong, uncomplaining
CENTAURY	Timid, anxious to please, submissive	OLIVE	Mental or physical exhaustion
CERATO	Distrust of self, easily led astray	PINE	Self-reproach, guilt, apologetic
CHERRY PLUM	Desperation, obsessive fear	RED CHESTNUT	Worry for others, imagining the worst
CHESTNUT BUD	Failing to learn from experience	ROCK ROSE	Sudden alarm, terror, panic
CHICORY	Possessive, attention-seeking	ROCK WATER	Self-denial, repression, perfectionism
CLEMATIS	Daydreaming, absent-minded, drowsy	SCLERANTHUS	Indecisive, unstable, unreliable
CRAB APPLE	Feeling unclean, self-disgust, tending to overemphasize small problems	STAR OF BETHLEHEM	Grief, shock, distress, past or present trauma
ELM	Occasional feelings of inadequacy, overwhelmed by responsibility	SWEET CHESTNUT	Utter desolation, extreme mental anguish, despair
GENTIAN	Easily discouraged, sense of doubt, despondency, negativity	VERVAIN	Overbearing, argumentative, fervent, fanatical
GORSE	Despair, hopelessness, resignation	VINE	Arrogant, domineering, ambitious
HEATHER	Self-centered, hungry for attention	WALNUT	Unsettled, undergoing transition
HOLLY	Anger, jealousy, hatred, revenge	WATER VIOLET	Aloof, retiring, self-reliant
HONEYSUCKLE	Nostalgic, homesick, living on memories	WHITE CHESTNUT	Persistent worry, preoccupation, internal arguments
HORNBEAM	Fatigue, lassitude	WILD OAT	Unfulfilled ambition, drifting
IMPATIENS	Irritability, impatience, dislike of constraint	WILD ROSE	Resignation, lack of interest, failure to make effort
LARCH	Lack of confidence, expecting failure, despondency	WILLOW	Bitterness, resentment, self-pity, lack of humor

Skin pain

P*roblems that affect the skin include eczema and psoriasis, both of which are known to be triggered by stress, among other things. Other painful conditions like blisters or a heat rash are caused by exposure to heat.*

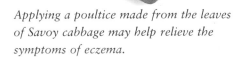

Eczema

Eczema is a widespread and sometimes severe skin condition, often caused by touching, eating, or drinking a substance the body reacts against. This is usually described as an allergic reaction, even though not all eczema is true allergy. Symptoms are intensely itchy, red skin that can become cracked, raw, and painful.

There are more than a dozen different types of eczema but the most common is atopic, or infantile, eczema seen mainly in children ("atopic" means having an inherited tendency). A vast range of substances can trigger eczema, but among the most common are detergents, dyes, plants, various foodstuffs, drinks, animal hair, feathers, and the mite, which is found in house dust.

People with eczema may often suffer from asthma as well, and there is a close link between these conditions and hay fever (usually a reaction to something breathed in such as house dust or pollen). Emotional stress is also a known trigger for both eczema and asthma (though not hay fever). A tendency to eczema is lifelong and there is as yet no cure, but a wide range of natural approaches can help keep this frequently distressing condition under control.

Applying a poultice made from the leaves of Savoy cabbage may help relieve the symptoms of eczema.

ACUTE ECZEMA TREATMENTS
Naturopathy

• For atopic eczema, rub on oil containing gammalinoleic acid (GLA), an essential fatty acid available in pharmacies and health food stores as evening primrose oil or starflower oil. Do not use skin creams containing lanolin.
• Bathe the affected area in 2 tbs of bicarbonate of soda (baking soda) dissolved in warm water.
• Apply a poultice of fresh Savoy cabbage leaves. Clean, warm, and crush the leaves before layering them on the affected area and bind them in place with a bandage. Repeat every night and morning.
• Apply calamine lotion, preferably containing arachis oil.
• Rub on essential oils of fennel, German chamomile, geranium, sandalwood, hyssop, juniper, rose, or lavender (12 drops to 3 tbsp carrier oil). If the affected area is dry, use calendula as a carrier oil;

if moist, use a neutral carrier such as grapeseed oil. Apply morning and night. Other oils said to help are almond oil and St. John's wort (hypericum) oil.

• Drink herbal teas of calendula (pot marigold), chickweed, walnut leaf, nettle, chamomile, and various berries (especially blackberry, raspberry, and loganberry).

• The dried herbs parsley, dandelion root, red clover, and goldenseal may also help. Mix with honey and use on bread as a spread. Goldenseal can also offer relief when an infusion is painted onto the skin: mix the dried herb with hot water and allow it to cool.

Homeopathy

The homeopathic remedies graphites, petroleum, *Rhus tox*, and sulfur are said to help relieve symptoms, but self-help is not recommended for eczema, particularly atopic eczema.

CHRONIC ECZEMA TREATMENTS
Dietary and nutritional therapies

Identifying and then eliminating allergens (substances that cause an allergic reaction) are the most important steps in the long-term treatment of eczema. Sometimes allergens are easy to identify—a reaction caused by animal fur, for example. If not, identification is normally done by an allergy test or, to identify allergens in food and drink, by an exclusion diet. Cut down on dairy products, eggs, animal fats, sugar, and salt. Avoid processed foods and those containing additives and preservatives. Eat more vegetables, vegetable oils, such as safflower oil, and oily fish such as tuna, mackerel, and herring. Whenever possible, eat organic foods.

Regular supplementation with gammalinoleic acid has had good results. The best known form is evening primrose oil but starflower (borage) and blackcurrant seed oils both contain high levels of GLA and all are widely available in pharmacies and health food outlets. The doses may need to be as high as six capsules a day and benefits may not become apparent for three months or so.

Other food supplements with a good record in helping control eczema over the long term (three months or more) are betacarotene (the natural precursor of vitamin A), vitamins B, C, and E, and the minerals zinc, selenium, and magnesium. ▶

Find out more	
Herbal medicine	60
Acupuncture	68
Homeopathy	70

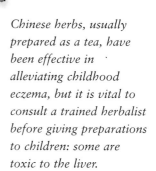

Chinese herbs, usually prepared as a tea, have been effective in alleviating childhood eczema, but it is vital to consult a trained herbalist before giving preparations to children: some are toxic to the liver.

CHINESE HERBAL MEDICINE

A "miracle cure" for atopic eczema was widely publicized in 1993 when a combination of 10 different Chinese herbs used by a Chinese herbalist in London appeared to have dramatic success with difficult cases. It was subsequently researched by a British company and patented under the name Zemaphyte after successful trials. Other traditional Chinese medical herbalists claim a similar success rate with different herbs from the range of over 4,000 herbs used in Traditional Chinese Medicine. Many Chinese herbs are extremely potent and not yet properly researched, however, so great care must be taken in choosing a fully qualified practitioner.

Skin pain

PSORIASIS

This condition is the result of skin cells reproducing at an abnormally high rate. It is a chronic skin disease that can develop on any part of the body, although it is usually seen on the head, lower back, knees, and elbows. It is characterized by dry, reddish patches covered with silvery scales that develop on the skin.

The underlying cause of psoriasis is unknown but there appears to be an inherited tendency which remains once it starts, flaring up and then abating at intervals. Attacks are classically triggered by stress and illness.

Psoriasis is neither infectious nor contagious and any pain experienced is usually psychological rather than physical —although severe forms can involve very painful cracks in the skin and, in very rare cases, a painful type of arthritis that affects the legs, hands, and spine.

TREATMENTS FOR PSORIASIS
Naturopathy

Natural sunlight contains ultraviolet A and B rays, and exposure has a beneficial effect on psoriasis. However, except in unusual places such as the Dead Sea (where the atmosphere contains vapors that filter the sun's rays), exposure must not be too long because the benefits will be outweighed by the dangers the sun poses to skin health.

Naturopaths recommend a mixture of fasting and juice therapy. Fasting for 48 hours (but no longer) can be done drinking only water or freshly pressed fruit and vegetable juices. If drinking only water, do not exercise and get plenty of rest. For a juice fast, carrot, celery, beet, cucumber, and/or grape are recommended, drunk as often as you want. This can be combined with moderate exercise.

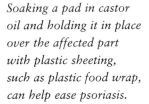

Soaking a pad in castor oil and holding it in place over the affected part with plastic sheeting, such as plastic food wrap, can help ease psoriasis.

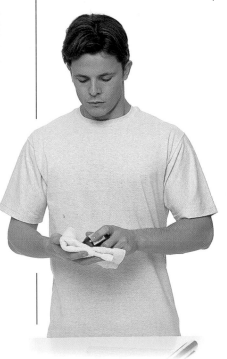
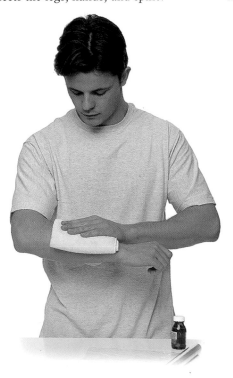
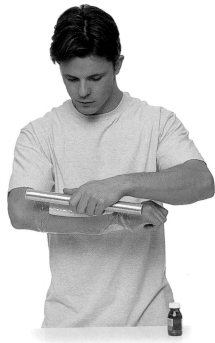

To encourage cleansing, take Epsom salts or castor oil in orange juice two days before starting the fast and the morning of the first day of the fast. Some naturopaths recommend castor oil packs and baths, as follows.

• **Pack:** Soak a cloth in castor oil so it is wet but not dripping. Apply to the affected area and cover with a plastic sheet. Place a heating pad on top, starting at medium heat and turning to high if tolerable. Leave the plastic on for 1–1½ hours and then remove and clean the skin with two teaspoons of baking soda in 3½ cups (1 liter) of warm water. Repeat four times a day.

• **Bath:** Fill a bathtub with warm water, adding half a cup of castor oil under the running water. Mix thoroughly. Soak in the mixture for 20–30 minutes, rubbing your body all over, and then wash it off with shampoo (the bathtub will be very slippery so be careful when standing).

Dietary and nutritional therapy

Eat a healthy diet, especially one with plenty of fresh fruit, vegetables, and salads, and reduce your intake of animal fats as much as possible. Oily fish such as mackerel, salmon, sardines, and herring are recommended. Bitter melon is an old remedy for psoriasis that might help, as well as avocado and sauerkraut.

Supplementing with a daily tablespoon of cold-pressed extra virgin olive oil, flaxseed (linseed) oil, or canola oil may help. Alternatively, take capsules of essential fatty acids (EFAs) containing gammalinoleic acid (GLA) and eicosapentaenoic acid (EPA), such as starflower (borage) oil, evening primrose oil, and fish oils.

Other supplements that might help during an attack are vitamin A (10,000 IU three times daily for six days), vitamin B-complex (100 mg twice a day with meals), vitamin D (400 IU a day), spirulina (an algae rich in micro-minerals), zinc (15–20 mg a day), and the tissue salts *silica*, *nat sulf*, *kali phos*, *ferr phos*, and *calc sulf*.

Herbal medicine

A type of berberis (*Mahonia aquifolium*) has recently shown success in treating psoriasis, but a more traditional treatment is dandelion root and burdock with red clover flower as blood cleansers. Nettle, too, is said to help psoriasis by purifying the blood. Other useful herbs are echinacea for the immune system, yellow dock (boil 2–3 leaves per quart of water and drink), garlic, and sarsaparilla.

Homeopathy

The remedies *sulfur* 6c (for dry, red, itchy patches), *petroleum* 6c (for dry, rough and cracked skin), and *graphites* 6c (for scaly patches that ooze) can help alleviate acute attacks of psoriasis. Take 3–4 tablets daily for 14 days.

Aromatherapy

The essential oils bergamot and lavender, added to bath water or rubbed on the skin via a neutral oil or lotion, may help.

Reflexology

Massaging the areas corresponding to the liver, kidneys, lungs, solar plexus, and diaphragm is said to help.

Mind–body therapies

Reducing stress and using relaxation techniques are important in preventing psoriasis. Approaches such as meditation, self-hypnosis, visualization, and biofeedback can all help. ▶

Find out more

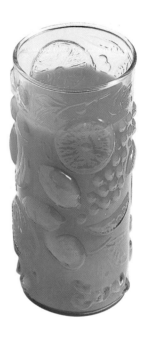

Naturopaths recommend drinking juiced vegetables to help alleviate psoriasis.

Skin pain

Protect a blister from infection by dabbing on an antiseptic essential oil before covering with a sterile dressing.

Common remedies for athlete's foot and related fungal infections include direct application of cider vinegar or, in severe cases, hydrogen peroxide (right).

BLISTERS

Painful, fluid-filled areas of raised skin, blisters are often caused when the skin rubs against a hard surface or by exposure to heat. They may also be the result of irritation, injury, inflammation, or a fungal infestation. Blisters are prone to infection if they burst or the skin is broken.

Herbal medicine

The natural antiseptics in lavender, tea tree, or Roman chamomile oils can be applied to a punctured blister to prevent infection and promote healing. (If you have to pop a contact blister, do so with a needle sterilized in a flame or an antiseptic solution.) Alternatively, apply a mixture of hypericum and calendula or rub in aloe vera gel. Adding garlic to your diet may also be helpful.

Homeopathy

Take the homeopathic remedy *Rhus tox* 6c every four hours for a day or take the tissue salt *Kali mur*.

HEAT RASH

An allergic reaction to too much heat or sun may result in a rash. It causes uncomfortable red blotches to appear over the surface of the skin. The more delicate the skin, the more susceptible the person—children and women seem to be more prone to heat rash than men.

The symptoms, though intense, are usually short-lived and disappear when the irritant is avoided.

Herbal medicine

Find somewhere cool and bathe the affected area with tincture of calendula (pot marigold) or lavender. Chamomile lotion or houseleek, applied with a cotton ball, will cool and soothe. Placing slices of cucumber on the rash is also soothing. A tea made from lime or peppermint may also help.

Aromatherapy

Apply a soothing mixture of one drop of sandalwood oil and 4 drops of lavender oil in 2 tbs of calendula carrier oil to the affected area.

Homeopathy

Take *Urtica* 6c, *Rhus tox* 6c or *Apis* 6c every 15 minutes for up to one hour, as necessary.

TINEA

This fungal infection of the skin is also, and misleadingly, known as ringworm—worms are not involved. It is most commonly experienced on the foot (as athlete's foot) but can also affect the groin and any other part of the body where warm, damp conditions may encourage the growth of fungi.

The most common symptom is intense itching but local pain may be felt if the condition is severe,

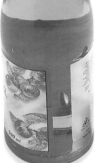
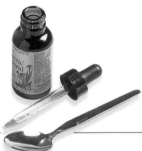

particularly between the toes if the skin is cracked and raw.

Keeping the affected area clean and dry is the most effective treatment so a high standard of personal hygiene is important. For athlete's foot, allow plenty of fresh air to get to the feet and wear cotton—never nylon—socks.

Herbal medicine

Among a number of treatments that can help when used on the affected area are propolis or calendula cream and vitamin C powder. Soaking a cotton ball in honey and cider vinegar and leaving it on the affected area overnight can also help.

A daily footbath of goldenseal root or a mixture of 1 oz (30 g) each of red clover, sage, calendula, and agrimony mixed with 2 tsp of cider vinegar is especially effective against athlete's foot. Bathe the feet for 30 minutes, dry well, and powder with arrowroot or powdered goldenseal root.

For severe cases, clean with a cotton ball soaked in hydrogen peroxide and follow with any of the treatments described above.

Aromatherapy

Undiluted tea tree essential oil applied to the affected area can help. For athlete's foot, add 2 drops each of essential oils of lavender, tea tree, and tagetes to a bowl of warm water and soak the feet for 10 minutes each night.

Alternatively, you can apply a compress of the same oils to the affected area at night and keep it in place until morning with a bandage or sock. In the morning, wash and dry the feet, apply a fresh compress using the same oils but add a tablespoon of calendula oil. Leave in place during the day.

BOILS

Inflammation of the skin as a result of a bacterial infection produces tender, pus-filled raised spots or boils. They usually appear on the face and neck but can also affect the rest of the body. They seldom clear unless the pus is drained first. Boils accompanied by fever and listlessness may require antibiotics as well as drainage.

Naturopathy

A hot poultice of slippery elm paste, kaolin, or magnesium sulfate can be applied for a few days to bring the boil to a head. After the boil has burst apply tea tree antiseptic oil.

An alternative is to make a bread poultice: crumble the bread into boiled milk or water, wrap it in gauze, and allow to drain. Apply while still hot. Do this every 3–4 hours. A hot Epsom salts pack, made with 2 tbs of salts to 1 cup of water, is also effective.

While the boil lasts, take 1 tsp of equal parts of echinacea, cleavers, and yellow dock made up as a tea. Drink three times a day.

Find out more	
Herbal medicine	60
Naturopathy	62
Homeopathy	70

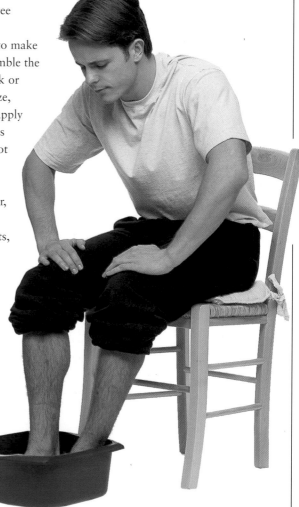

A daily herbal footbath can help ease the symptoms caused by athlete's foot.

Head pain

*A*lmost everyone has experienced head pain, ranging from *relatively transient conditions such as headaches, toothaches, and sore throats to more debilitating ones, such as migraines and tinnitus. A number of complementary therapies can help.*

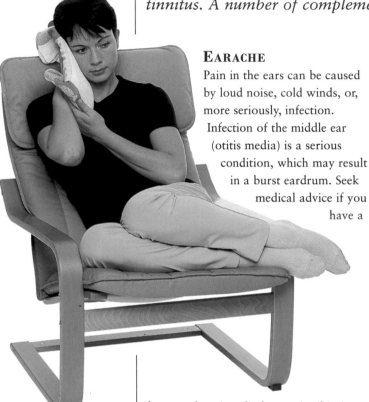

Naturopaths recommend applying heat to the ear in the form of a covered hot water bottle. This improves the circulation to the area and may help to relieve the pain.

EARACHE

Pain in the ears can be caused by loud noise, cold winds, or, more seriously, infection. Infection of the middle ear (otitis media) is a serious condition, which may result in a burst eardrum. Seek medical advice if you have a fever or there is a discharge. Antibiotics may be advisable. Nothing should be introduced into a discharging ear.

Naturopathy

If the pain recurs, reduce your intake of dairy products, drink 6–8 glasses of water a day, and cover your ears in the wind. Regular supplements of vitamin C, zinc, and garlic can also help.

Herbal medicine

Put 2–3 drops of warmed almond or castor oil into the ear and seal with a cotton ball. You can also try oil drops of garlic, St. John's wort, or mullein.

Alternatively, place 2 drops of tinctures of pennywort, chamomile, yarrow, hyssop, or lobelia in the outer ear, protected with a cotton ball plug. Or try a hot onion or mustard poultice placed behind the ear until the ache eases.

If infection is the cause of the ache, use echinacea tincture every 2 hours: take 30 drops (half a teaspoon) for an adult, or half that dose for a child.

Homeopathy

If the ears have a discharge, take *Hepar sulf* 3c. If an earache follows an infection, take *Silicea* 12. For the early stages or recurrent earache, take *Ferrum phos* 3c/6c or *Aconite* 3c. If the face is flushed, take *Belladonna* 3c. For restlessness and irritability, take *Camomilla* 3c, and if these feelings follow measles or whooping cough, take *Pulsatilla* 3c.

TINNITUS

Usually described as a ringing, buzzing, hissing, roaring, or whistling, tinnitus is a

WARNING

If you suffer from persistent head pain consult your doctor. It can signal conditions which need immediate medical attention:
- *Cancer*
- *Cerebral hemorrhage*
- *Concussion*
- *Meningitis*
- *Poliomyelitis*
- *Stroke or aneurysm*

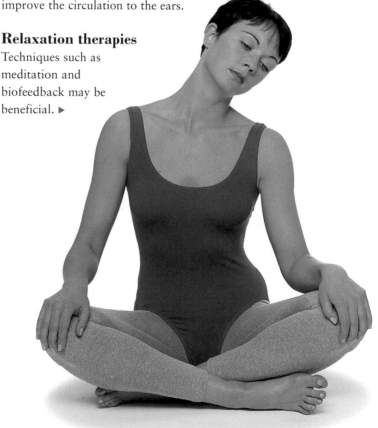

A traditional Native American remedy, ear candles clear the ear and may be helpful for alleviating tinnitus.

constant background noise in the ear. It tends to be depressing to the emotions rather than painful. Persistent tinnitus should be investigated by a doctor; it may be a symptom of another illness. Tinnitus may be due to diseases of the inner ear or the nerves supplying the ear. Other causes include depression, stress, anxiety, infection, high blood pressure, drugs, and congestion with wax.

Naturopathy

Inhaling steam containing the same herbs that can clear noses and sinuses can help (see Sinusitis, p. 104).

Herbal medicine

Ear "candles" are thin hollow tubes, containing herbs that are placed in the ear and slowly burned down to the ear.

The heat creates a vacuum that draws wax and other impurities into the tube, and the smoke from the burning herbs is said to have a healing effect on the ear. It takes about 10 minutes to do one ear. The technique is simple and painless but it is best to have help.

The herb ginkgo biloba may also help, taken either as a capsule or as a tincture of equal parts with black cohosh. It may take some time to be effective.

Acupressure

Locate the acupressure point on top of the cheekbone, about a finger's width from the ear. Press for a few seconds and release. Alternatively, press the web of the hand between the thumb and index finger.

Homeopathy

For pain with giddiness and a roaring noise, seek medical advice to rule out serious problems, then take *salicylic acid* 6c; if there are ringing, tinkling, or hissing noises, take *Cinchona* 6c. Other remedies are *Carbon sulf* and *Kali iod*. It is best to consult a qualified homeopath.

Yoga

Head and neck exercises can help improve the circulation to the ears.

Relaxation therapies

Techniques such as meditation and biofeedback may be beneficial. ▶

Find out more	
Acupressure	38
Yoga	40
Homeopathy	70

Slowly rotating the head and trying to touch your shoulders with your ears is a yoga exercise that helps alleviate the symptoms of tinnitus.

CHAPTER THREE

Head pain

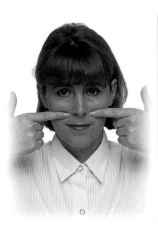

Pressing the acupressure points located on the sinuses can help ease the symptoms of sinusitis.

SINUSITIS
Sinusitis is inflammation and infection of the sinuses, and produces phlegm. Colds or the flu may also initiate acute sinusitis, which may lead to bacterial infection. Chronic sinusitis can be as painful as a severe migraine—and as hard to clear.

Naturopathy
Steam inhalation with eucalyptus and/or pine oil (or, for a stronger effect, menthol) will help alleviate the immediate symptoms. Gargling and washing the nasal passages with a teaspoon of salt in warm water can help clear congestion. Take supplements of vitamins C and B-complex and zinc.

Acupressure
Pressing the points shown in the picture *(left)* can help relieve sinus pain. Or try the point, "Liver 4" on the web of the hand between thumb and first finger.

Massage and aromatherapy
As an alternative to acupressure, massage the whole area of the nose, eyes, cheekbones, and temples with a mixture of essential oils of peppermint (9 drops), eucalyptus (6 drops), and lavender (10 drops) in 25 drops of carrier oil.

Herbal medicine
A tea of equal parts echinacea, golden rod, goldenseal, and marsh mallow leaf is effective drunk every two hours. Garlic, horseradish (raw or in capsules), and echinacea (tincture or capsules) also help.

Dietary therapy
Prevent attacks by avoiding dairy products, bananas, peanuts, coffee, alcohol, and hot, spicy foods. Try to determine if there is an allergic cause for the phlegm.

Practitioner therapies
• Acupuncture

HAY FEVER
More properly called seasonal allergic rhinitis, hay fever is an allergic reaction to a number of environmental factors, particularly pollen and dust. This results in inflammation of the lining of the nasal passages, causing sneezing, runny nose, itchy and weeping eyes, and a sore throat.

Naturopathy
Wash the nasal passages with a little salt in warm water and take supplements of vitamin C with bioflavonoids (natural antihistamines) and vitamin B-complex.

Herbal medicine
Drink a cup of tea 2–3 times a day made from two parts elderflower to one part each of ephedra, eyebright, and goldenseal.

A month before the hay fever season starts (in spring to early summer), take 0.5–1 tsp of tincture of licorice in warm water twice daily.

Acupressure
Pressing the point in the webbing between thumb and first finger can help.

Homeopathy
To help relieve itching eyes and sneezing, try *Arsenicum album* 6c, *Sabadilla* 6c, and *Allium cepa* 6c.

EYE STRAIN
Reading, working at a computer screen for long periods of time, and watching too much television all prevent the eyes from blinking as frequently as normal. This can lead to dry eyes. Strain can occur if the vision is weak and the eyes may "weep" under excessive strain.

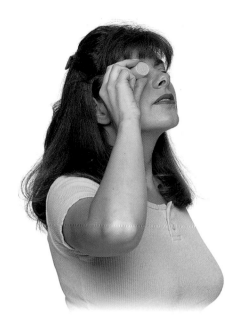

Bathing the eyes with Euphrasia, also known as eyebright, is an effective remedy to ease tired eyes.

Massage and aromatherapy

Massaging the neck and shoulders with lavender or neroli oil diluted in a carrier oil of almond or grapeseed is beneficial.

Herbal medicine

Bathe the eye with eyebright, either using an eyebath or soaking a cotton ball in the liquid and applying it to your eyes for 20 minutes every hour while the pain lasts. Other useful plants are chickweed, calendula, and cucumber. For severe eye strain, grate a raw potato and place enough on the closed eyelid to cover the whole eye. Cover with gauze and leave for 1–2 hours.

Homeopathy

Try *Arnica* 6c for tired eye muscles; *Natrum mur* 6c if eyes are aching; *Ruta grav* 6c if eyes feel as if they are burning or if you experience strain after reading.

CONJUNCTIVITIS

Inflammation of the membrane inside the eye tissue is known as conjunctivitis, or pink eye. It causes redness, pain, and often a sticky discharge. Infection is usually the cause, so medical advice should be sought, unless it is very mild. Other causes include an allergic reaction or irritation caused by smoke and chemical sprays.

Herbal medicine

Wash the eye several times a day with a mixture of one tablespoon of goldenseal root powder, one teaspoon of salt, and 250 mg vitamin C. Add 3½ cups (1 liter) of clean water and mix well. Let the mixture settle before using.

Homeopathy

Bathe the eye three times daily in one part *Euphrasia* tincture to 10 parts boiled water and take 5 tablets of *Ferrum phos* 6c dissolved in hot water four times a day. Other helpful remedies, all at 6c, are *Belladonna*, for the early stages of inflammation; *Aconitum*, for severe pain with itching and blistering; *Apis mel*, for burning, sensitive eyes; *Euphrasia*, for stickly lids; *Mercurius corr* for discharging itchy eyes; and *Pulsatilla nigricans* for hot, watery eyes. If symptoms recur, consult a qualified homeopath. ▶

Find out more	
Aromatherapy	36
Acupressure	38
Homeopathy	70

EYE EXERCISES

Blinking rapidly followed by "palming" can help strained eyes. To palm, rub your hands together vigorously to generate heat and then place both hands over the eyes while breathing deeply. Hold them there for several minutes. Some people also find gazing at a lighted candle helps.

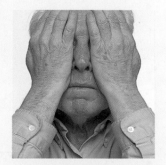

Head pain

Swilling the mouth with diluted hypericum can help ease the pain that persists after a tooth extraction.

TOOTH ABSCESS

Also known as a gumboil, an abscess is a small, pus-filled boil in the root of the tooth. Treatment is almost always required from a dentist or dental surgeon, who will drain the pus – to relieve the pain and swelling – or remove the tooth. Antibiotics will be prescribed to control the infection. Care has to be taken to ensure that the pus does not enter the blood stream, from where it may be carried to other tissues.

While waiting for your dental appointment, try one of the following remedies to help ease the pain – which can be considerable.

Naturopathy

An ice pack held to the face over the sore area can help to bring relief. To make your own, wrap a bag of frozen vegetables in a dish towel.

Homeopathy

Start with *Belladonna* 200c every hour, followed with *Silicea* when the abscess has been drained. *Hepar sulph* 30c or 200c is recommended for less severe pain. Again, once the abscess has been drained, follow this with *Silicea*. *Hypericum* 30c and hypericum tincture diluted in warm water and used as a mouthwash can also help with the pain experienced after a tooth extraction.

Herbal medicine

After dental work, rinse the mouth with a mouthwash made from half calendula tincture and half hot water. Do not take calendula if you are pregnant or breastfeeding, unless specifically advised to do so by a medicinal herbalist.

FACE AND JAW PAIN

Face pain may be caused by toothache, by inflammation of the nasal and sinus cavities or by neuralgia. Jaw pain may be the result of an emotional or psychological problem, as well as a physical one. Teeth-grinding and clenching the jaw are frequent causes of jaw pain, as is poor tooth alignment, a poor bite or even badly fitting dentures.

Jaw pain can also be due to posture problems such as the head being held at an awkward angle, or habitually standing or sitting with the jaw jutting forward. This can produce increasing strain on the hinge joint between the jawbone and the skull – the temperomandibular joint – and its attaching ligaments. This type of pain is usually known as TMJ tension for short. Depending on its cause, TMJ tension may respond to rest and painkillers, but there may be strain on the jaw muscles which hurt – or may even lock – whenever you open or close your mouth. The jaw may also "click" or "pop" and severe headaches may result.

Naturopathy

A covered hot-water bottle makes an effective hot compress for face pain as a result of inflammation of the nasal and sinus cavities. For face pain caused by toothache, a cold compress made with a pack of frozen peas is effective (see also Toothache, p. 111).

For TMJ pain, alternating hot and cold compresses using either of the above techniques may provide some relief. But if the problem is long term, it may require

Find out more

Naturopathy	62
Homeopathy	70
Neuralgia	130

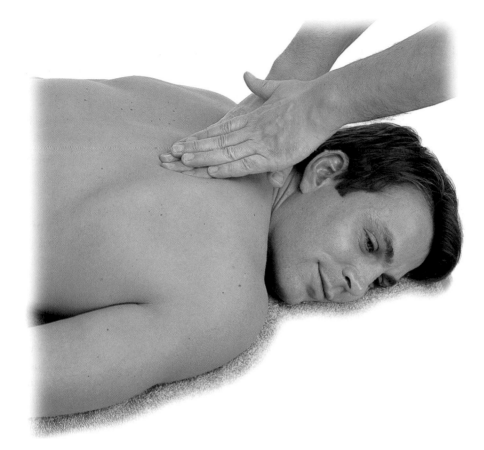

Massage eases the muscles and helps you to relax. This in turn, relieves face and jaw pain caused by tension and awkward posture. Basic massage techniques are not difficult to learn and can bring great physiological and psychological benefits.

treatment by a specialist in musculo-skeletal correction, such as an osteopath or chiropractor (see pp. 64–67), or a teacher of the Alexander technique (see p. 66).

For face pain caused by nasal inflammation, see the remedies suggested for sinusitis on page 104.

Relaxation therapies

As tension is often a major factor in face and jaw pain, therapies that help relax the face muscles and joints can be highly effective. Among those that have proven effective are meditation (see pp. 48–49), biofeedback (see p. 47), autogenic training (see p. 51), yoga (see pp. 40–42) and massage (see pp. 56–57)

with one or more of the relaxing essential oils (see pp. 36–37). Lavender oil is excellent for muscle aches, as well as stress; rosemary is effective for muscular aches and strains.

Practitioner therapies

- Cranial osteopathy
- Acupuncture

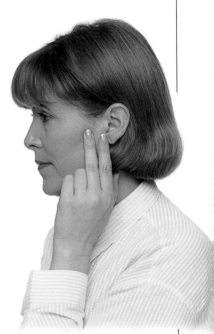

There are 45 acupressure points along the stomach meridian, one of the body's 12 meridians. The point to relieve TMJ pain is Stomach 7, located about a thumb's width in front of the ear. Press this point for about a minute.

Head pain

SORE THROAT

Also known as pharyngitis, a sore throat is caused by the inflammation of the pharynx, the area at the back of the mouth. The term "sore throat" is also applied to inflammation of the adenoids, tonsils (tonsillitis), and the voice box or larynx (laryngitis).

Laryngitis causes a sore throat, characterized by hoarseness and loss of voice. If there is no obvious cause for these symptoms, such as from shouting or singing too loudly, a sore throat is often the first sign of either bacterial or viral infection, which may be an additional symptom of a cold or flu. Prompt and early action can help prevent the infection from becoming more serious.

Nutritional therapy

Take vitamin C with bioflavonoids, zinc, vitamins A and E, and fish oil (EPA) to boost immunity.

Herbal medicine

Gargling provides instant symptomatic relief for a sore throat, whatever the cause. Dilute sea salt in warm water or cider vinegar, honey, and lemon. You can also use sage, thyme, propolis, echinacea, or spilanthas. Chewing licorice root or sucking slippery elm tablets will also help.

Garlic, either eaten raw or taken in capsule form, and echinacea extract boost immunity. Teas of marsh mallow, plantain, elderflower, and catmint alleviate symptoms and promote recovery.

Homeopathy

Try *Belladonna* 30c , *Hepar sulf* 6c, *Mercurius* 6c, *Arsenicum* 6c, or *Apis mel* 6c for inflammation and pain. For tightness, try *Lachesis* 6c, *Lycopodium* 6c, or *Phytolacca* 6c.

TONSILLITIS

Tonsillitis is inflammation of the tonsils. It is sometimes caused by a virus but is more commonly due to an infection, usually one of the streptococcus bacteria. Symptoms are a very sore, red, swollen throat, fever, headache, swollen neck glands, and sometimes a dry cough.

Recurrent infection damages the tonsils by building up scar tissue. It may also lead to the formation of an abscess, known as a quinsy, around the tonsil. The throat threatens to close completely and prevent breathing. If this happens, seek immediate medical help.

Naturopathy

Bed rest and taking plenty of fluids are recommended, especially diluted fruit juices and warm broths or light soups. Solid foods are not necessary for the first 48 hours.

Herbal medicine

Gargle with tea made from a teaspoon of powdered ginger, which will also promote sweating. Pure, undiluted tincture of goldenseal sprayed onto the tonsils with a small spray will promote rapid healing. Drinking powdered root of licorice dissolved in warm water will relieve any coughing. An alternative remedy is gargling with, and then swallowing, a tea of 1 oz (30 g) of fresh sage, or a cup of hot water mixed with a few drops of grapefruit seed extract.

Homeopathy

For infected, painful tonsils, difficulty in swallowing, and discharge, try *Merc sol* 30c. For pain and fever with bad breath, use *Mercurius* 30c. For a sudden attack with fever, swelling and a red and stiff neck, use *Belladonna* 30c.

When taking dosages, take one tablet every hour for 12 hours, followed by one dose three times daily for two days. However, an individual prescription from a homeopath is advised for cases of recurrent tonsillitis, especially those affecting children.

Note: Antibiotics are advisable in cases of severe bacterial (but not viral) infection, particularly in children. To replace the healthy bacteria destroyed by antibiotics, you should take a course of acidophilus or bifidophilus with plain, live yogurt to restore natural gut flora. ▶

COLDS AND THE FLU

Colds and the flu produce a variety of uncomfortable symptoms.

In colds, symptoms are mainly confined to the head, particularly in the ears, nose, and throat. Most colds go away after about a week or so, with or without treatment.

The flu can be felt throughout the body, especially in the joints, chest, and lungs. One of the most elusive viral illnesses, the flu is more serious than a cold and requires bed rest, at least in its preliminary stages.

Natural therapists insist that the symptoms of colds and the flu should not be suppressed, particularly if there is a raised temperature. Instead, the fever should be encouraged to come out by promoting sweating.

Individual symptoms can be treated as indicated elsewhere in the book, but the following approaches will also help accelerate recovery.

NATUROPATHY
Rest, keep warm, and drink plenty of fluids (6–8 glasses a day), particularly if you are suffering from a raised temperature and sweating. Mix honey and lemon, or cider vinegar, in hot water and drink regularly. Frequent inhaling of proprietary mixtures such as Olbas oil (containing eucalyptus,

juniper berry, menthol, clove, wintergreen, cajuput, and mint oils) helps clear nasal passages and eases breathing difficulties. Either sprinkle the mixture on a handkerchief or make it into a steam inhalation.

NUTRITIONAL THERAPY
Take vitamin C with bioflavonoids (3–5 g a day), zinc (15–20 mg a day), vitamin B-complex (best as a multivitamin, with iron), and cod liver oil (EPA). If you feel hungry (although loss of appetite is normal and aids recovery), eat lots of fresh fruit, nuts, seeds, whole grains, and fresh vegetables.

HERBAL MEDICINE
Echinacea, garlic, ginger, and lemon can help combat infection (take echinacea as either a tincture or capsule). Drink hot tea made of equal parts of yarrow, elderflower, and peppermint at least three times a day. Add boneset if you have a fever.

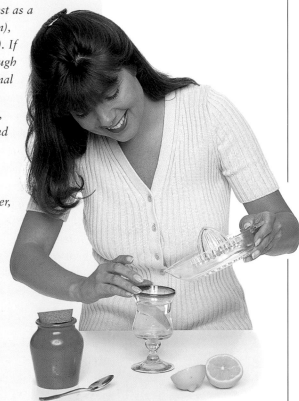

Head pain

CANKER SORES

Painful canker sores are likely to be caused by a combination of factors, particularly stress, a depleted immune system, bad diet, and nutritional deficiency. The virus that triggers cold sores (see below) can sometimes cause canker sores, as can accidentally biting your inner cheek or wearing badly fitting dentures.

See your dentist or doctor if canker sores do not clear up within two weeks.

Herbal medicine

Rub aloe vera gel on to the sore. A mouthwash of calendula, myrrh, and thyme will also help. Alternatively, mix clove and tea tree oil with glycerine and apply it to the canker sore.

Nutritional therapy

Take a good multivitamin and mineral supplement containing vitamin B-complex, vitamin C, and zinc to help recover from or prevent canker sores.

Practitioner therapies

• Homeopathy (individual prescription from a trained homeopath is essential)

COLD SORES

The virus *Herpes simplex* I causes these highly contagious blisters. After the initial infection the virus lies dormant in the body until triggered into action by various causes such as stress, too much sun, colds or the flu, a lowered immunity, or high temperature. Some are lucky enough to experience only the first, initial attack, while others regularly have outbreaks of the painful sores. A variation on the same virus (*Herpes simplex* II) causes genital herpes.

Rubbing an ice cube on a cold sore is a simple remedy that helps to reduce discomfort.

If you have a cold sore you should avoid physical contact with others—particularly kissing—while the sore is still moist. Even using the same towels or pillowcases can spread the infection.

To avoid transmission of the virus, wash immediately if you touch the affected area or are touched by someone who has an outbreak. Take particular care not to transfer the infection to the eyes.

See a doctor immediately if sores do emerge near the eyes—they can be painful and may cause eyesight problems unless treated early.

Naturopathy

In the early, more painful stage an ice cube used intermittently on the sore can reduce the pain. Lemon juice diluted in cold water and applied can also help. Alternatively, vitamin E cream or vitamin E oil can be applied to the affected area.

Dietary and nutritional therapies

Eat a healthy diet with as much fresh fruit, vegetables, live unadulterated yogurt, and fiber as possible. Avoid sugar, refined foods, and alcohol.

Take supplements to boost the immune system, particularly vitamins A, C with bioflavonoids, E, and B-complex. Also take zinc, selenium, magnesium and calcium, lysine, and acidophilus.

Herbal medicine

Licorice root has antiviral qualities, said to be effective against the herpes virus.

GUM PAIN

Pain in the gums is usually the result of a buildup of plaque around the base of the teeth, which causes inflammation there, a condition known as gingivitis. It is often brought about by poor tooth and gum care, especially inadequate brushing and flossing.

The gums become sore and bleed and, in extreme cases, the teeth may begin to loosen and fall out.

Naturopathy

Regularly rub the gums with lemon juice, salt, or bicarbonate of soda and rinse out. Follow this application with an herbal mouthwash (see below).

Herbal medicine

Essential oils of tea tree, lavender, geranium, or thyme can be applied to the gum to ease the pain.

Use a mouthwash of the tinctures of calendula, myrrh, and wild indigo or St. John's wort in warm water. Toothpaste containing aloe vera can also help.

Homeopathy

Rhus tox, Hepar sulf, or *Nat mur* may help. Start with a 30c or 6c dose every 4 hours for 2 days and then every morning and evening for 3 days. If bleeding from the teeth is heavy, take one tablet of *phosphorus* 30c every 10 minutes and then hourly, as necessary.

TOOTHACHE

A toothache can be extremely painful and you will need to see a dentist to check if the tooth root or gum are infected or defective in some way. Temporary alleviation of pain is possible with the following remedies.

Herbal medicine

Soak a cotton ball in oil of cloves, which has natural anesthetic properties, or cinnamon oil, peppermint extract, or alcohol. Dab it around the sore area. Alternatively, chew a clove on the area.

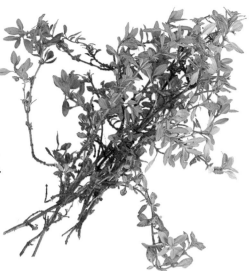

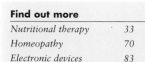

Gum pain can be calmed by dabbing essential oil of thyme directly on the affected area.

The herbs white willow bark and meadowsweet are natural painkillers but are best taken as tablets.

Naturopathy

An ice pack held to the face over the sore area can help bring relief.

Homeopathy

Try *Conitum* 3c for throbbing and/or burning pain; *Chamomila* 3c or 6c for nerve pain, especially in children; or *Pulsatilla* 6c or *Calcarea phos* 6c for pain with tearfulness.

Pain-relieving devices

TENS and intrasound devices (see p. 83) can help alleviate a toothache. Treatment needs to last 45–60 minutes.

Practitioner therapies

• Acupuncture

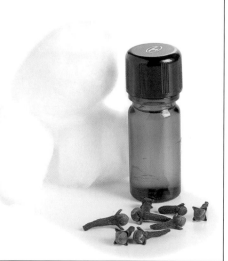

A cotton ball soaked with oil of cloves and placed on the tooth is an effective way to ease any pain.

Head pain

HEADACHE

The most common and widely experienced pain is headache. It is also the most common type of referred pain.

Most headaches are tension or nervous headaches caused by tightness in the muscles and tissues of the head, neck, and shoulders, usually from the stresses and strains of everyday living. Other common causes of headaches are overeating and excessive alcohol consumption, which produces the characteristic hangover.

These types of common headache are fairly easy to treat. Headaches caused by more serious conditions such as infection, allergic reaction, or inflammation are harder to treat but help is still possible.

Prolonged or frequent aches and pains in the head should be reported to a medical practitioner.

Naturopathy

Naturopathy uses hydrotherapy to treat the immediate symptoms of tension headaches and a variety of relaxing techniques to remove the underlying causes. For immediate relief, soak a compress or face cloth in cold water, wring it out, and lie down or sit comfortably. Place the cold compress over your closed eyes and forehead, resting for as long as possible. Resoak and wring out the cloth as often as needed to keep the head cool and ease the headache.

Aromatherapy

For headaches caused by colds, the flu, or breathing problems such as sinusitis and bronchitis, steam inhalations can be effective. Pour a few drops of an essential oil, such as eucalyptus, juniper berry, peppermint, wintergreen, and cajuput, into a bowl of very hot water. Cover your head with a towel and breathe in the vapor for about 5 minutes.

A relaxing alternative is to soak in a hot bath to which you have added melissa, rosemary, or marjoram oils.

Acupressure

Using both hands, apply gentle fingertip pressure to a point midway between the eyebrows and another immediately above

HOMEOPATHIC REMEDIES FOR HEADACHE

Homeopathic remedies can be a useful first-aid treatment in emergencies, but most homeopaths would advise a consultation with a qualified homeopath rather than self-prescription, particularly for recurring or chronic headaches. If you are pregnant, don't take any remedies without advice.

CAUSE OF HEADACHE	REMEDY	DOSE
OVEREATING, FEELING BLOATED	*Pulsatilla*	6c, one every hour until better
INDIGESTION, CONSTIPATION	*Nux vomica*	6c, one every night and morning
FEAR, EMOTIONAL EXCITEMENT	*Gelsemium or Ignatia*	6c, one every hour until recovered
HEAT EXPOSURE, SUNSTROKE	*Belladonna*	6c, one every hour until better
INJURY OR FALL	*Arnica*	6c, one every hour until better

on the top of the head. Hold the pressure for about 5 seconds and then relax. Another point to press is the web between thumb and first finger (do not do this during pregnancy).

To ease a tension headache, place the tips of your middle fingers in the hollows at the base of the skull on either side of your neck. Press firmly for a minute.

Relaxation therapy

Consciously getting your body to relax and noting the change helps to prevent and remove headaches caused by tension in other parts of the body. Deep breathing will help calm the mind and ease tension headaches (see pp. 48–49).

Massage

Sit in a comfortable position (in a hot bath is ideal) and massage the back of the neck, shoulders, and temples. Use relaxed but firm strokes on the shoulders, and fingertip pressure on the back of the neck and temples. This is even more effective if you lubricate your fingers and hands with a neutral oil such as grapeseed and add 3–4 drops of lavender, basil, or chamomile essential oils. Massaging the temples with peppermint oil or menthol can also help. You can also try inhaling these oils.

Reflexology

In reflexology the toes are said to relate to the head, so apply firm fingertip or thumb pressure to the bottom, sides, and top of the toes of both feet. Concentrate on any areas where the toes are tender, pressing until the soreness or tenderness wears off. Do the same to the area where the toes join the foot, which is said to correspond to the neck. If you suffer from recurring headaches, it might be worth consulting a professional reflexologist.

Herbal medicine

You might try meadowsweet and the bark of the willow tree. These contain natural painkillers that can ease headaches—aspirin was developed from them.

Other useful herbs for combating headaches include valerian, chamomile, passiflora, ginger, lavender, and rosemary. They can be taken as a tea by pouring hot water on to 1–2 tsp of the dried herb. Allow the herbs to infuse for a few minutes before drinking.

Healing and therapeutic touch

Get a friend or partner to stand behind you and stroke your temples with their hands placed about 1 in (2.5 cm) away from your hairline.

Ask your partner to wish or will your headache away as they stroke. Visualize the headache going away while this is happening. Do this for about 10–15 minutes or as long as it takes to be effective.

Practitioner therapies

- Alexander technique
- Cranial osteopathy ▶

Find out more	
Aromatherapy	36
Relaxation	46
Homeopathy	70

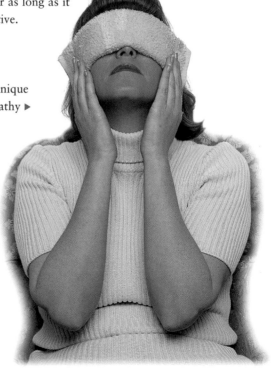

To ease a headache, sit quietly with a cool compress or towel over your eyes and forehead.

Head pain

MIGRAINE

A severe and often disabling pain in the head, usually on one side only, is known as a migraine. Sometimes it is accompanied by alarming symptoms, such as altered perception, a feeling that the skull is in the grip of a tightening vice, pins and needles, or numbness in the limbs, nausea, vomiting, and an inability to do anything.

Symptoms can come and go and may last for several hours, sometimes even days. No two people experience identical symptoms and different symptoms can be experienced on different occasions, so migraines are notoriously difficult to treat.

Prolonged or frequent aches and pains in the head should always be reported to a medical practitioner.

Herbal medicine

The herb feverfew is known to be effective in preventing attacks, particularly for migraines relieved by warming the head. One fresh leaf a day (in a salad or sandwich) is recommended if you are prone to regular bouts,

although is is not as effective once an attack has started. Alternatively, take feverfew in 125 mg capsules or tablets every 4 hours.

Dietary and nutritional therapies

Beneficial foods include carrots, celery, beets, cucumber, spinach, and parsley. For best effects they should be juiced.

Supplements of vitamin C, the B vitamins (especially vitamin B_3), and the mineral magnesium are said to help prevent attacks and alleviate the symptoms. Take them in a good-quality multivitamin or consult a qualified nutritional therapist for optimum doses. Royal jelly is also said to be effective.

Acupressure

A number of pressure points are effective, depending on the symptoms. The majority are on the upper back, shoulders, and the back of the neck, so it is best to ask someone to help you. They should apply gentle but constant pressure for about 10 seconds. Repeat for as long as is

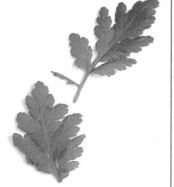

Feverfew is an herbal remedy that has been used for centuries to ease migraines and headaches.

MIGRAINE AURAS

Migraines, which have been compared to something like an electrical storm going on inside the head, seem to have many causes. The most common are extreme stress, disco lights, noise, menstruation (women suffer from migraines much more than men), and eating or drinking trigger foods such as chocolate, cheese, oranges, coffee, and red wine.

Migraine auras are hallucinations caused by chemical disturbances in the brain. They can be felt visually—as

stars, flashing lights, zigzag patterns, or blank spots in your field of vision—but also as a change in the other senses of hearing (music that isn't there, for example), taste, smell, and touch. Some people experience changes in their sense of reality or perception. Even speech and memory can be affected. This can be so severe that it can leave sufferers feeling very disorientated.
Warning: Prolonged or frequent aches and pains in the head should be reported to a medical practitioner.

MAKING WAVES

A device developed in the UK in the 1980s that makes use of low-level electromagnetic waves is claimed to have a success rate of around 80 percent in reducing the incidence of migraines. (This is not, however, borne out by controlled trials.)

The device, invented by electronics engineer and migraine sufferer Steven Walpole, gives out minute electro-magnetic impulses every few seconds to correct the deficiency in the sufferer's brain waves that is said to cause the migraine. For example, correcting a

deficiency in the theta brain waves, which are involved in pain control, reduces pain. The device is small enough to be worn as a watch or pendant, but in order to be effective it must be specially programmed by a trained practitioner using a computerized brain-frequency analyzer.

Available in Europe, North America, South Africa, and Australia under the brand names Trimed *and* Empulse, *the device is claimed to relieve other aches and pains, including back pain, arthritis, sciatica, and allergic reactions.*

comfortable or until the migraine fades. Be careful not to overstimulate the point because this may aggravate the symptoms for a short period.

Reflexology
As for headaches (see p. 113).

Massage and aromatherapy
Massaging the head, neck, shoulders, back, feet, and hands can sometimes bring relief. Some people, however, do not like to be touched during a migraine attack.

The massage should be soothing instead of vigorous. Use long, smooth strokes. Continue as long as is comfortable and until it brings relief. If trying aromatherapy, use the same oils as for headaches (see p. 112).

Relaxation therapies
Meditation, t'ai chi, and yoga help with the long-term prevention of migraines because they encourage the body to relax and "balance" itself.

Homeopathy
For acute attacks take an hourly 6c dose of *Nat mur, Lycopodium, Nux vomica,* silica, or spigelia. However, self-help is not usually recommended for migraines because effective treatment depends on circumstances and symptoms.

Self-hypnosis
The technique of warming the fingers by using the power of your mind has been shown to produce lasting benefits for many sufferers of chronic migraine. The technique, which is a form of self-hypnosis, involves willing your fingers to reach a temperature of 96°F (35.6°C). It is said to work for 85 percent of people.

Practitioner therapies
- Acupuncture
- Counseling and psychotherapy
- Hypnotherapy
- Osteopathy and chiropractic

Drinking the juice of root vegetables, such as carrots and beets, and green ones including spinach, and celery, may ease a migraine attack.

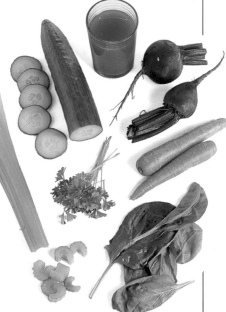

Chest and lung pain

A part from coughs, which may be more irritating than serious, most chest and lung ailments need careful monitoring. Bronchitis, pneumonia, pleurisy, asthma, emphysema, and tuberculosis should all be treated by qualified practitioners of both conventional and complementary medicine.

BRONCHITIS

Bronchitis is inflammation of the bronchi, the tubes that connect the windpipe to the lungs. It is caused by viral and bacterial infections. Symptoms include coughing, wheezing, phlegm, shortness of breath, and tightness in the chest, often with a headache and fever.

Acute bronchitis will usually clear with treatment in about 10 days but chronic bronchitis is harder to clear and can be extremely serious, requiring specialist medical attention.

A course of antibiotics may be necessary for severe cases of bacterial (not viral) bronchial infection.

Warning: Bronchitis can be a serious illness; seek medical attention.

Naturopathy and aromatherapy

Bed rest in a warm room is advisable in the early stages of infection. Avoid airway irritants such as smoke and dust.

Steam inhalations provide the quickest form of relief—try 5 or 6 drops of essential oils of eucalyptus, hyssop, cedarwood, or sandalwood. Many other essential oils can help various symptoms of bronchitis, so consult a qualified clinical aromatherapist.

A warming compress can remove tightness and soreness in the chest.

Dietary and nutritional therapies

Avoid dairy products, sugar, and eggs; they are mucus-forming. Eat hot, spicy foods instead to loosen the mucus.

Try an all-juice diet for the first two to three days of an infection. Good choices are blends of carrot and radish; carrot, beet, and cucumber; or carrot and spinach. Drinking plenty of liquids is more important than eating in the first 48 hours.

Take supplements of vitamins A, B-complex, C with bioflavonoids, and E, as well as the minerals zinc and selenium.

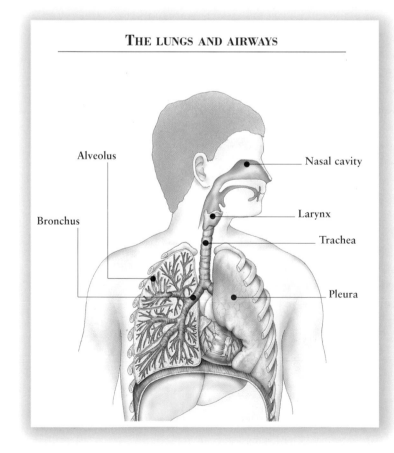

THE LUNGS AND AIRWAYS

Alveolus

Nasal cavity

Bronchus

Larynx

Trachea

Pleura

Herbal medicine

Fresh garlic or garlic capsules and echinacea can help prevent and fight infection. Teas of elecampane, licorice root, and ginger can clear mucus and are warming. Take three times a day, hot or cold as preferred. There are more than a dozen herbs effective for bronchial infection, so the advice of a qualified medical herbalist is necessary to treat individual symptoms.

Homeopathy

The remedies *Bryonia, Aconite,* sulfur, phosphorus, *Arsenicum alb,* and *Pulsatilla* are recommended for various symptoms, but an individual prescription is advised.

Reflexology

Manipulate the front part of both feet, from the arch to the toes. Concentrate on those parts that feel tender, working on them until the tenderness goes.

COUGHS

Coughing is the body's natural way of expelling any substance that interferes with breathing and usually resolves itself when the cause of the problem (such as dust or smoke) is removed. However, coughing caused by an infection such as the flu, or inflammation in the respiratory tract, such as laryngitis or bronchitis, can be painful and needs treatment to clear.

See your doctor if the coughing lasts for more than two weeks without improving, or is accompanied by pains in the chest, a high temperature, and blood in the mouth.

Naturopathy

A hot drink of lemon juice, honey, and glycerine is a good throat soother. A hot apple-cider vinegar compress wrapped around the throat and upper chest can help loosen phlegm.

Dietary and nutritional therapies

Take a garlic capsule 2–3 times a day. Also take a daily multivitamin tablet that includes betacarotene (vitamin A), B-complex, C, and zinc.

Herbal medicine

White horehound is the best of a wide range of herbs that help alleviate coughs. Others are mullein, wild lettuce, yarrow, angelica, elecampane, licorice, and elderflower. For children, wild cherry bark is good. Make a tea and drink a spoonful three times a day. A number of herbal cough mixtures available from health food stores contain a mixture of most of the herbs known to be effective.

Aromatherapy

Steam inhalation with various essential oils such as eucalyptus, cypress, hyssop, bergamot, or chamomile is beneficial, especially in the early stages. Inhale for about 10 minutes using 3–4 drops of the chosen oil in very hot water. Massaging the chest and back with the diluted oils of eucalyptus, thyme, sandalwood, frankincense, or myrrh can also help.

Acupressure

Pressing a point on the back by the heart, between the spine and shoulder blade, can relieve muscle spasms caused by coughing. Ask someone to hold the pressure for about 5 seconds and repeat as needed.

Homeopathy

Remedies include *Bryonia, Aconite, Pulsatilla, Rumex,* and *Arsenicum alb.* ▶

Find out more

Nutritional therapy	*33*
Herbal medicine	*60*
Reflexology	*74*

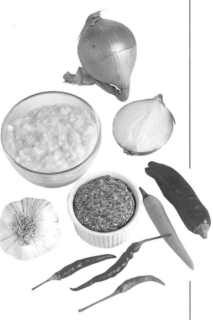

Hot foods, such as chilies, onion, mustard, and horseradish, are excellent decongestants. Dairy products, in contrast, are mucus-forming and should be avoided if you suffer from respiratory illnesses.

Chest and lung pain

PNEUMONIA

Pneumonia is an infection of the lungs (either one or both) caused by a virus or bacterium. Symptoms are chest pains, breathlessness, a cough with colored phlegm, fever, and chills. Bacterial pneumonia is more serious than viral. Bronchopneumonia is often the final stage in people dying of old age and cancer and is sometimes a feature of acquired immune deficiency syndrome (AIDS).

Warning: Pneumonia can be life threatening. Immediate treatment with antibiotics is advisable in cases of bacterial pneumonia. See your doctor.

Naturopathy

Rest and various hydrotherapeutic methods are recommended, including a warming compress covering both the back and chest (also known as a pneumonia jacket). This should be combined with the application of a cold compress to the forehead, with the feet in a bowl or basin of hot water. The treatment should be followed by having someone beat on the back with cupped hands to loosen mucus in the lungs and (in normally strong people only) finished with a cold friction rub.

Dietary and nutritional therapies

Eat plenty of fresh fruit and vegetables (include raw garlic, chili, and cayenne peppers) and avoid dairy produce and sweet foods. Fresh diluted pear juice is claimed to have decongestant qualities and regular drinks of fresh juiced carrot, spinach, parsley, garlic, and cumin are said to help. Take supplements of large daily doses of vitamins A (preferably in the form of betacarotene), C with bioflavonoids (6–10 g), and zinc. Other useful supplements are propolis (bee pollen) and acidophilus/ bifidophilus (probiotics).

Pneumonia and pleurisy affect the lungs. Massaging the back helps ease lung pain.

Herbal medicine

Lobelia and thyme help to loosen phlegm; echinacea and garlic fight infection; and elderflower and yarrow reduce fever. They should be taken as teas made from the dried herb or tinctures.

Other useful herbs are ipecacuanha, hypericum, and juniper. Get an individual prescription from a qualified herbalist.

Massage and aromatherapy

Massage the back and chest with equal number of drops of essential oils of camphor, eucalyptus, pine, lavender, lemon, and tea tree diluted in a carrier oil.

Reflexology

As for bronchitis (see p. 117)

Practitioner therapies

- Acupuncture
- Osteopathy
- Homeopathy

PLEURISY

When the pleura, the membrane between the lungs and the walls of the chest, becomes inflamed, pleurisy results. The most usual cause is a viral infection but it can be brought about by pneumonia and injury or inflammation of the heart and lungs. Breathing produces sharp, stabbing pains in the chest and shoulders from the fluid buildup in the membranes and there may also be a high fever.

Warning: Pleurisy can result from a serious disease such as cancer or a pulmonary embolism. Medical advice is essential.

Naturopathy

Rest and drink plenty of fluids. Hot compresses applied to the back and chest will bring relief and promote recovery.

Diet and nutritional therapies

Hot soups and broths, especially if they contain the spices turmeric, garlic, and cloves, and chewing the rind on the inside of citrus fruits can all help soothe the pain of pleurisy. Drinks of juiced carrot, celery, and parsley (or carrot and pineapple; or carrot, beet, and cucumber) can also be beneficial. "Toast water," a traditional remedy of powdered whole-wheat toast boiled in water with butter and salt, and drunk while warm, is said to relieve pleurisy pain.

Taking the supplements vitamin C (2–3 g), vitamin A (50,000 iu), EFAs (fish oils, starflower/evening primrose oils), and bromelain (pineapple enzyme) may also aid recovery.

Herbal medicine

Mix equal parts of the tinctures of pleurisy root, echinacea, and elecampane and take a spoonful a day.

Drinking a tea of equal quantities of dried mullein and pleurisy root as often as needed during the day can also help.

Massage and aromatherapy

Massaging the back and chest with the oils of black pepper, pine, myrrh, rosemary, angelica, sage, or tea tree is effective in reducing fluid buildup.

Reflexology

As for bronchitis (see p. 117)

Practitioner therapies

- Acupuncture
- Homeopathy

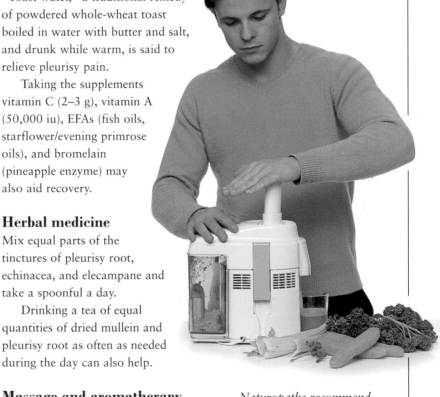

Naturopaths recommend drinking juiced vegetables to ease the symptoms of pneumonia and pleurisy.

Chest and lung pain

ASTHMA

This recurrent chronic breathing problem is caused by constriction of the bronchi and bronchioles (the breathing tubes), which produces attacks of wheezing and breathing difficulty. It is often due to an allergy, though irritation of the lining of the bronchi and broncioles can also produce an attack.

Childhood asthma often clears when adolescence is reached, but adult asthma is usually chronic. A number of therapies help alleviate symptoms and promote recovery.

Foods rich in magnesium, betacarotene, and antioxidants may protect the lungs. If you feel an attack coming on, drink raw fresh fruit and vegetable juices, including grapefruit, celery, spinach, and carrot.

Warning: Severe attacks of asthma are potentially life-threatening. Immediate medical help must be sought, especially if the sufferer develops blue lips and cold, clammy skin during an attack.

Naturopathy

The naturopathic approach focuses on identifying and removing the cause(s) of the allergic reaction and supporting the immune system to help deal with them. Identifying allergens can be difficult. Food allergens can be identified by following an exclusion diet but environmental allergens are harder to isolate. Recent research makes the house dust mite—found in pillows and bedding—the leading culprit.

Ionizers and humidifiers may help if breathing is affected by air conditions. Alternating hot and cold foot baths, dry skin brushing, and mustard or hot mud packs on the chest may also help.

Dietary and nutritional therapies

Identify food allergens by keeping a daily diary of what you eat, then follow your findings with an exclusion diet, preferably aided by a dietitian.

Eating a healthy diet and avoiding known allergens, such as dairy products, food additives, and colorings is a priority. Raw juice diets are recommended, particularly carrot, celery, spinach, and grapefruit, or radish, lemon, garlic, carrot, horseradish, and beet. Cider vinegar with honey in a glass of warm water taken three times a day can also help.

Nutritionists may advise supplements of propolis (bee pollen), omega-3 and omega-6 essential fatty acids, vitamins A (or betacarotene), C, E, and B-complex, and minerals magnesium, calcium, selenium, and manganese.

TESTS FOR ASTHMA AND ALLERGIES

Testing for allergies is still a far from exact science. A variety of tests is available that claim to identify allergens—substances that cause allergies—and they include blood tests, electrical tests (Vega and MORA), muscle tests (applied kinesiology), and pulse tests. Experts do not regard any of them as reliable because they are not based on recognized scientific principles, have not been fully researched and tested, and they rely too much on the subjective judgement of the tester.

New tests are constantly being devised, however, and favorable test results indicate that a reliable test may soon be available.

COMMON ASTHMA TRIGGERS

- *House dust*
- *Animal dander (fur, hair, skin)*
- *Pollens and seeds*
- *Weather (very dry, very cold air)*
- *Air pollution (vehicle fumes, tobacco smoke, mold)*
- *Stress*
- *Exercise*
- *Food additives*
- *Viral infection*
- *Medicines and drugs*

Herbal medicine

An herbalist may recommend ephedra (*Ma huang*), ginseng, euphorbia, chamomile, elecampane, or thyme to ease breathing. Mullein, marsh mallow, butterbur, slippery elm, and passionflower soothe and clear the mucus membranes. They are taken as either tinctures or teas.

Warning: It is essential to visit a fully trained herbalist for a professional prescription if you have asthma or any other serious condition.

Massage and aromatherapy

Essential oils of bergamot, camphor, eucalyptus, lavender, hyssop, and marjoram are recommended for an attack. Mix two drops of each oil into a carrier oil and massage gently over the back and chest. To help mucus drain, lie with the head slightly lower than the lungs while the massage is performed. Eucalyptus, juniper, wintergreen, peppermint, and rosemary are also suitable. For asthma attacks brought on by stress, essential oils of lavender or frankincense are said to be calming.

Acupressure

Relax the neck, letting the head drop onto the chest. Press the point on the front of the shoulder where it joins the chest for two minutes, with the thumbs (*see picture, below*). Breathe slowly and deeply while doing this.

Psychological therapies

Stress and anxiety can trigger an attack or worsen an existing attack. Mental relaxation exercises such as visualization, meditation, and biofeedback can help.

Alexander technique/yoga

Alexander technique and yoga exercises help the chest expand fully.

Reflexology

As for bronchitis (see p. 117)

Practitioner therapies
- Osteopathy
- Cranial osteopathy
- Homeopathy
- Acupuncture/Traditional Chinese Medicine
- Psychotherapy
- Hypnotherapy

Find out more	
Acupressure	38
Visualization	50
Herbal medicine	60

Acupressure points that may help for lung problems are located on the front of the shoulder, below the collar bone.

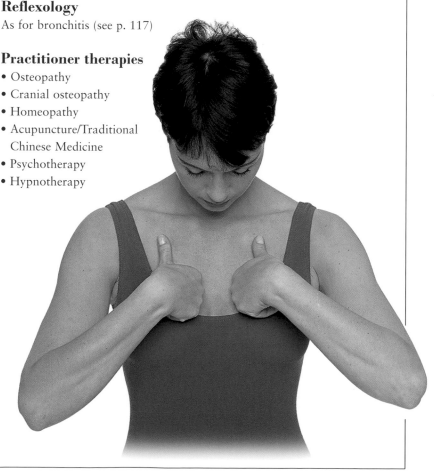

Chest and lung pain

EMPHYSEMA

This progressive disease of the lungs occurs when the tiny air sacs (alveoli) that transfer oxygen breathed from the air into the bloodstream become damaged. They fail to work effectively, causing increasingly severe breathlessness. Damage is usually caused by smoking or prolonged exposure to polluted air but sufferers of chronic bronchitis and asthma can also be affected.

Although, as yet, emphysema is incurable, there are effective self-help treatments to ease symptoms. These include gentle exercise such as swimming, t'ai chi, and yoga, using ionizers and humidifiers, and back patting with cupped hands (see p.57).

Dietary and nutritional therapies

Eat hot, spicy foods such as garlic, chili peppers, mustard, horseradish, and onions. Avoid mucus-forming dairy products such as milk, cream, and cheese to ease congestion. Drink juiced fruit or vegetables to fortify the body's defenses. Combinations of garlic, celery, spinach, watercress, carrots, potatoes, barley, and wheatgrass; and blackcurrants, oranges, lemons, and grapes can help. Supplements of vitamins A, B-complex, C, and E, as well as co-enzyme Q10, zinc, and lecithin are recommended.

Herbal medicine

Drinking tea made from licorice root may help ease an attack.

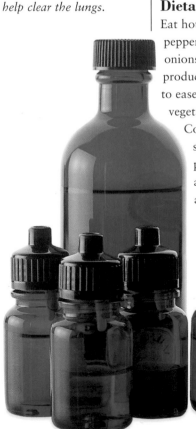

Aromatherapy oils, used either as part of a massage or inhaled with steam, can help clear the lungs.

Massage and aromatherapy

Massaging with essential oils of cedarwood, pine, peppermint, and eucalyptus, or inhaling steam with basil, cajuput, eucalyptus, hyssop, or thyme oil will help ease the lungs.

Relaxation techniques

Biofeedback, meditation, and visualization can aid relaxation (see pp. 46–54).

Reflexology

Applying pressure to the reflex points corresponding to the lungs can help if done on a regular basis (see pp. 74–75).

Practitioner therapies

- Acupuncture
- Osteopathy
- Chiropractic
- Homeopathy

TUBERCULOSIS

A severe bacterial infection, tuberculosis (TB) is a caused by the organism *Mycobacterium tuberculosis*. It is a systemic disease and so can affect any part of the body including the brain, lymph glands, small intestine, kidneys, and bones. Usually, however, it affects the lungs. Symptoms include pain, fatigue, breathlessness, loss of appetite and weight loss, fever, night sweats, and coughing blood. From a low between 1944 and 1985, the incidence of the disease has risen in recent years.

Immunization with the BCG vaccine remains the preventive treatment of choice among doctors but it is not widely known that BCG is only partly effective in some people. It is not a blanket remedy. Moreover, immunization limits diagnosis in cases of suspected tuberculosis because once vaccinated, a person will register permanently positive in standard tests.

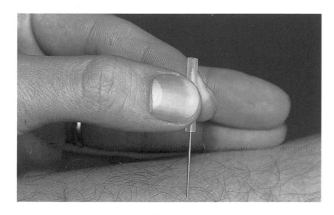

Acupuncture needles have rounded ends that part the flesh so they do not cause any pain when they are inserted. Acupuncture may relieve the pain associated with lung complaints.

Warning: Tuberculosis is a potentially fatal illness; seek medical advice if you are suffering from any of its symptoms or have been in contact with a sufferer.

Dietary and nutritional therapies

Fresh fruit, particularly grapes, bitter melon, and pears, and raw vegetable diets with garlic are recommended. Drinking a mixture of equal portions of raw potato and carrot, juiced with a little olive or almond oil and honey, and taken three times a day is said to be beneficial. Allow the potato liquid to settle and then skim off the starch before using.

It is also important to eat foods such as milk, eggs, fish, and meat to maintain protein intake.

Supplements that may be useful to strengthen the system include vitamins A, B-complex, C, and E, the minerals zinc, calcium, and magnesium, both omega-3 and omega-6 essential fatty acids from fish oils, and GLA from evening primrose and starflower oils.

Naturopathy

The clear, dry air found in mountain areas is very much part of the original naturopathic treatment. If this is not practical, try to rest in the sunshine and fresh air whenever possible.

A hot pack of eucalyptus oil and alcohol applied to the chest can help clear the lungs.

Short fasts are recommended, but only under a trained naturopathic therapist's supervision.

Herbal medicine

Echinacea is a potent booster of the immune system and is especially effective if taken as a tincture with mullein and elecampane. Take a teaspoon 3 times a day with food. Citrus seed extract and licorice root are also beneficial.

Massage and aromatherapy

Massaging the chest and back can help ease breathing problems and stimulate the body's natural defense mechanism. Massage is especially effective if done with essential oils diluted in a neutral carrier oil. Try eucalyptus, ginger, neroli, tea tree, cypress, rosemary, juniper, marjoram, or peppermint.

Practitioner therapies

- Acupuncture
- Chinese herbal medicine
- Homeopathy
- Osteopathy
- Psychotherapy
- Hypnotherapy

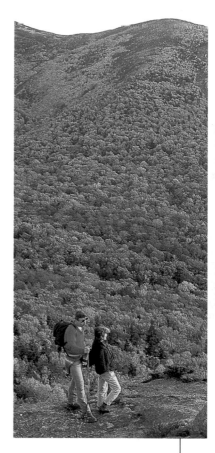

Clean, fresh mountain air is part of the traditional treatment for tuberculosis.

CHAPTER THREE

Heart and circulation pain

CHILBLAINS

Caused by a combination of extreme cold and poor circulation, chilblains appear as reddish-blue swellings that itch and burn. They usually occur on the hands and feet. If you have been exposed to extreme cold, seek medical advice to rule out frostbite, in which tissue loss can occur.

Naturopathy

Mix the white of an egg and a tablespoon of flour with glycerin and honey, work it into a paste and spread it over the affected part (do not rub). Cover with a cloth or bandage and leave for 24 hours.

Foods rich in vitamin E such as seeds, nuts, wholegrains, green leafy vegetables and wheatgerm (or supplements) and the herb echinacea can also aid recovery.

Homeopathy

For burning, itching and inflamed skin, apply *Rhus tox* cream twice daily. Take agaricus muscaria every 3 hours or *Carbo veg* if chilblains feel worse in a warm bed. For split, cracked skin, apply *Tamus* ointment and *Petroleum 6c* three times daily for two weeks.

POOR CIRCULATION

Aches and pains in parts of the body other than the heart is occasionally the result of poor or interrupted circulation. The hands, legs and feet are commonly affected. Medical advice is necessary, since interruption may lead to tissue death.

Poor circulation anywhere in the body can be helped by diet, regular cardiovascular exercise, and stress reduction.

The "Mediterranean" diet, which includes plenty of fresh fruit and vegetables, fish, garlic and a little red wine, is beneficial to the cardiovascular system.

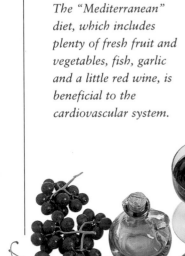

Dietary and nutritional therapies

Healthy eating advice applies particularly strongly for every condition involving the heart and arteries. Along with a "Mediterranean" diet (see picture left), onion, ginger, chilli peppers and alfalfa seeds have all been shown to aid circulation if eaten regularly.

Taking supplements of antioxidant nutrients also have proven benefits. The main ones are the vitamins A, C and E; the minerals selenium, zinc and magnesium, the amino acid lysine; the essential fatty acids EPA (from fish oils) and GLA (from starflower and evening primrose oils); and lecithin. There are now many proprietary formulas on sale with the correct doses.

Herbal medicine

Many herbs are said to help poor circulation, particularly to the extremities. The most popular are ginkgo biloba, hawthorn (*Crataegus*), cayenne pepper, lily of the valley, buckwheat, lime blossom, dandelion and broom.

Yoga

The postures known as the shoulder stand and the fish (see right) are said to be particularly beneficial for circulatory problems in the extremities, as well as for the digestive and respiratory systems. If the shoulder stand is too difficult, the less demanding half-shoulder stand can be equally effective.

Practitioner therapies

• Artery stretching is a highly specialized form of acupressure widely practiced in Japan. Though effective, it can be dangerous in untrained hands, particularly for those with advanced arterial diseases.

Warning: These yoga postures are not recommended for those with high blood pressure or those who have been diagnosed as having a heart condition. They are also not advisable during menstruation and should not be performed by anyone with eye, ear or brain infections. See the specific warning for shoulder stands below.

Be sure to check with your medical practitioner before attempting them if you have any doubts. ▶

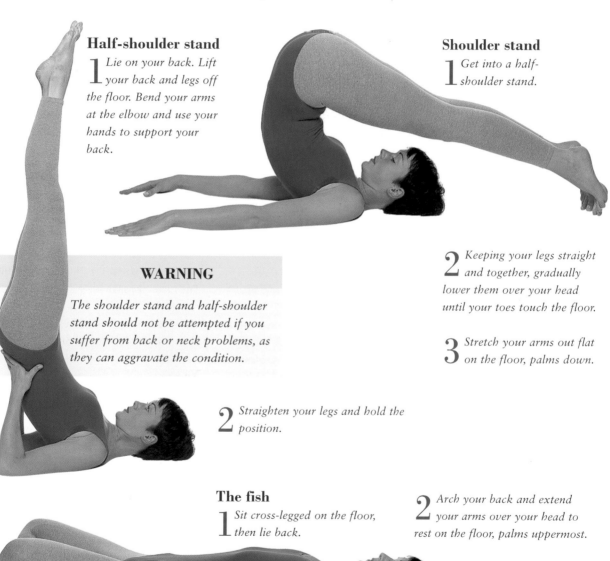

Half-shoulder stand

1 *Lie on your back. Lift your back and legs off the floor. Bend your arms at the elbow and use your hands to support your back.*

Shoulder stand

1 *Get into a half-shoulder stand.*

2 *Keeping your legs straight and together, gradually lower them over your head until your toes touch the floor.*

3 *Stretch your arms out flat on the floor, palms down.*

WARNING

The shoulder stand and half-shoulder stand should not be attempted if you suffer from back or neck problems, as they can aggravate the condition.

2 *Straighten your legs and hold the position.*

The fish

1 *Sit cross-legged on the floor, then lie back.*

2 *Arch your back and extend your arms over your head to rest on the floor, palms uppermost.*

Heart and circulation pain

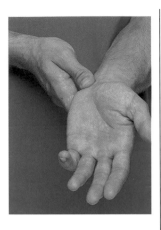

To ease palpitations, press the acupressure point on the wrist crease, on the tendon that attaches to the little finger.

The network of veins carrying blood around the body is prone to inflammation if circulation is poor, resulting in chilblains, varicose veins, and piles. The heart, at the center of the system, can also be affected by conditions such as angina and palpitations.

ANGINA

Known medically as angina pectoris, this condition causes pain in the heart muscle, usually as a result of poor circulation in the arteries that supply the heart muscle with blood.

Lifestyle advice is essentially the same as for all heart and arterial problems: exercise, diet, and stress reduction coupled with emotional support.

Warning: Although new thinking suggests that angina may not always lead to a heart attack, medical advice is vital to ensure that the pain is, in fact, angina.

Dietary and nutritional therapies

Healthy eating advice applies particularly strongly for every condition involving the heart and arteries. Eat salads, fish, garlic, red wine, vegetables, and fruit.

Taking regular supplements of antioxidant nutrients has been shown to have both preventive and recuperative benefits. The main ones are the vitamins A, C, and E; the minerals selenium, zinc, and magnesium; the amino acid lysine; the essential fatty acids EPA (from fish oils), GLA (from starflower and evening primrose oils); and lecithin.

Herbal medicine

Garlic, bromelain, lime blossom, lily of the valley, motherwort, and hawthorn berries (*Crataegus*) all have a reputation for removing angina symptoms completely over the long term. However, it is advisable to consult a qualified

herbalist in order to establish the correct dose for each person.

Drinking yarrow tea can also help. Make an infusion with 2 teaspoons of dried herb and drink three times a day.

PALPITATIONS

Palpitations are rapid and/or irregular heartbeats. The anxiety they cause can often be more serious than the physical problem itself. Palpitations can have a psychological cause such as worry or panic, although they are just as likely to be the result of an infection or having eaten and drunk something, such as tea, coffee, alcohol, and certain prescription drugs, that brings on an attack.

Relaxation techniques

Slow, deep breathing and biofeedback techniques help aid relaxation.

Homeopathy

To help during an angina attack, take *Aconite 6c*. This can help control and shorten the attack.

Acupressure

Treatment is on a heart point, located below the pisiform bone on the wrist, which is below the little finger.

Herbal medicine

Chronic attacks benefit from valerian and hawthorn berry in the form of tablets. An infusion of lemon balm, lime blossom, motherwort, or passionflower is beneficial if taken regularly.

PHLEBITIS

Inflammation of the veins, usually in the legs, is described as phlebitis. It is linked to varicose veins (see p. 128), although it may occur at the site of an injection.

Although painful, phlebitis is usually harmless and normally passes on its own. However, always seek medical advice, since complications may result. Effective treatment is simply to raise the leg. Elasticated stockings and similar supports can help.

Herbal medicine

Natural anti-inflammatories and painkillers such as willow bark and meadowsweet will help ease the pain.

RAYNAUD'S DISEASE

A painful condition, Raynaud's disease causes the small arteries of the fingers and toes to go into spasm, and the hands and feet to go cold, numb, and white. It is associated with chronic exposure to vibration, such as pneumatic drills. A similar intermittent problem, Raynaud's syndrome is usually associated with exposure to cold, and affects mainly young women.

Dietary and nutritional therapies

Iron-rich foods, such as liver, chicken, dark green leafy vegetables, soybeans, and black kidney beans, can help, as can multivitamin and mineral supplements containing vitamins C, E, and B-complex, along with copper, iron, and selenium.

Caffeine-rich drinks, such as coffee and tea, constrict blood vessels and reduce iron absorption, so are best avoided. Smoking also impairs circulation by constricting the blood vessels and causing hardening of the arteries.

Biofeedback

Learning biofeedback techniques enables you to improve circulation by controlling muscular tension. ▶

Find out more	
Acupressure	38
Biofeedback	47
Herbal medicine	60

Elevating the leg is the simplest and most effective way of easing pain caused by phlebitis, but make sure that there is no pressure on the calf. Avoid prolonged resting, which may lead to deep vein thrombosis and pulmonary embolism.

Heart and circulation pain

VARICOSE VEINS

Varicose veins are small pockets of congestion in the blood vessels that contain "used" blood—blood returning to the heart and lungs for reoxygenation. Varicose veins are caused by poor circulation. The veins show as lumps that can be both painful and itchy and may lead to phlebitis (see p. 127).

Women suffer far more than men, with pregnancy being a common cause. Other causes are not getting enough exercise, standing still for long periods, and being overweight.

Naturopathy

Alternating hot and cold compresses on the affected area (starting with the hot compress) can alleviate pain and improve circulation.

Dietary and nutritional therapies

Drinking combinations of vegetable juices is said to be effective for varicose veins. Try the following: carrot, celery, and parsley; carrot, celery, and spinach; carrot, spinach, and turnip; or carrot, beet, and cucumber. Juiced watercress on its own may also help. As part of a diet, raw beet, apricots, cherries, rosehips, blackberries, and buckwheat are all said to be beneficial.

Taking supplements of vitamins C (500 mg) and E (400 IU), along with rutin and lecithin is advised.

Herbal medicine

Hawthorn berries (*Crataegus*), horse chestnut, ginkgo biloba, and the bark or berries of prickly ash may be effective. Qualified herbalist advice is required.

Aromatherapy

Do not massage over affected veins. Instead, use a few drops of the oils of

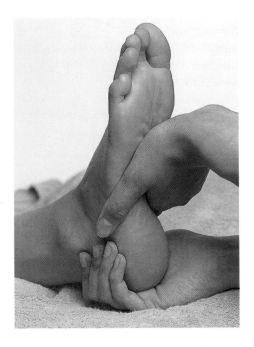

A general reflexology massage to the feet is said to be of benefit for varicose veins. Therapists may concentrate on more specific areas.

cypress, lemon, lime, or sandalwood in a warm (not hot) bath to ease pain.

Reflexology

Therapists claim that massaging the web between the second and third toes of both feet can benefit circulation.

Yoga

Practice the shoulder stand and the fish postures (see p. 125).

HEMORRHOIDS

Hemorrhoids are a type of varicose vein that forms at the opening of the anus, often as a result of recurring constipation and straining to evacuate. The veins become distended and enlarged and often rupture, causing pain, irritation, and bleeding during bowel movements.

Warning: You should seek medical advice immediately if bleeding continues for more than 12 hours or if there is no obvious cause for the bleeding.

Naturopathy

Ice packs applied to the affected area can bring immediate relief, but bathing in alternating hot and cold water is recommended for the longer term.

Sitz bathing, in which the feet are placed in cold water while the bottom is in hot water, and vice versa, is the ideal treatment, but this is only really practical at health spas with such facilities. An alternative remedy you can try at home is to have a warm bath with 1 lb (500 g) of sea salt added or three or four drops of essential oils of cypress and/or chamomile. Soak in the bath for up to 10 minutes. Regular cardiovascular exercise, such as brisk walking or cycling, helps overcome poor circulation and so will help avert another episode. You can also try yoga.

Dietary and nutritional therapies

Eat a healthy diet of fresh fruit and vegetables with plenty of whole foods to provide fiber. Drink at least 6–8 glasses of fresh water daily or try diluted fruit juice between meals. Take a large daily spoonful of flaxseed (linseed) oil.

Taking supplements of vitamins C (500 mg) and E (400 IU), along with rutin and lecithin is advised. If bleeding is heavy, take a good multivitamin tablet with iron.

Herbal medicine

Apply peony ointment to veins protruding from the anus and peony suppositories to those inside. Dab witch hazel on a cotton ball onto hemorrhoids that are bleeding. Other effective herbal ointments include calendula, St. John's wort, pilewort, comfrey, horse chestnut, and yarrow.

Yarrow can also be drunk as a tea or applied as a compress to relieve symptoms. To make a compress infuse 1–2 tsp of dried yarrow in a cup of hot water for 10 minutes. Dip a clean cloth into the infusion and apply to the affected area until the cloth is cold.

Movement therapies

Lie with the legs at a 45° angle to a wall for 3 minutes a day.

Practitioner therapies
• Homeopathy

Find out more	
Dietary therapy	30
Yoga	40
Naturopathy	62

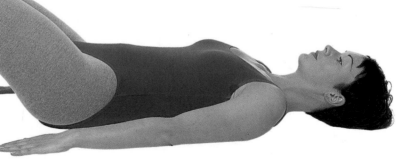

To ease hemorrhoids, lie on your back on the floor with your legs up at a 45-degree angle. Support your feet by resting them against a wall.

Musculoskeletal pain

B*ack problems and arthritis between them account for a high percentage of the pain experienced in the western world. Symptoms range from muscular spasms to inflamed joints. Nerve pain is characterized by aching and tingling but there may be stabbing or burning pain, too.*

Fresh vegetables are essential to good health. Eat raw or lightly steamed to retain as many nutrients as possible, or try juiced as an alternative to fruit juice.

NEURALGIA, NEURITIS, AND SCIATICA

Among the most common nerve problems are neuralgia (meaning pain from a nerve, particularly in the face), sciatica (pain from the sciatic nerve, which runs from the lower part of the spine down each leg), and neuritis (inflammation in any nerve). These pains can be caused by a number of physical and psychological factors; the most common are infection, poor posture, poor diet, stress, and overexertion.

Post-herpes neuralgia often follows an attack of shingles. The pain, which can be quite intense, results from damage to nerve endings, and it can persist for several months, particularly in people over 50 years of age.

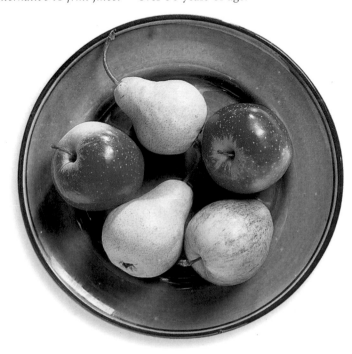

Naturopathy

Alternating ice and hot packs helps to relieve pain and promote recovery. Use a bag of frozen peas and a covered hot-water bottle, as often as needed.

Bathing in water at body temperature (a "neutral bath") is very soothing. Yoga and swimming are also helpful, especially combined with a sauna or steam bathing.

Diet and nutritional therapies

Eat plenty of green vegetables and fresh fruit. Including oats in your diet may also be beneficial.

You should also take the following supplements: vitamins A, C, E, and B-complex; the minerals magnesium, calcium, and selenium; omega-3 and omega-6 fatty acids (fish oils, linseed/flaxseed oil, and starflower or evening primrose oil). A good-quality multivitamin and mineral supplement contains most of these. Bromelain, an enzyme extracted from pineapples, is a natural nerve anti-inflammatory. Take up to 3 g a day between meals.

Herbal medicine

Regularly drinking teas of ginseng, hops, Jamaican dogwood, pasque flower,

If a food allergy or intolerance is implicated in causing nerve pain, a cleansing fruit or vegetable juice fast of no more than 48 hours may be beneficial. Common combinations are apple and pear, and beet and carrot.

passionflower, St. John's wort, skullcap, and valerian is recommended for nerve pain. Extract of black cohosh (*Cimicifuga racemosa*) is a natural anti-inflammatory.

Garlic milk—two crushed garlic cloves in 1 cup (250 ml) of milk—drunk daily can help sciatic pain.

Homeopathy

Neuralgia can be helped by *Belladonna* 6c and *Aconite* 6c; nerve injuries by *Hypericum* 6c. Take once an hour for up to 4 hours. *Bryonia* and *Rhus tox* may help to ease the pain of sciatica, but it is always advisable to consult a qualified homeopath for individual prescription.

Massage and aromatherapy

Massaging painful areas with two drops each of the essential oils of wintergreen, peppermint, and myrrh can help. You could also try rosemary and lavender, or clove, basil, and eucalyptus oils.

St. John's wort (hypericum) oil is also beneficial if rubbed into the affected area.

Acupressure

For facial pain, press a point on the inner end of the eyebrow on the side of the pain or points on either side of the mouth.

For sciatica, press on the outside of the bottom part of the leg a hand's width (including the thumb) from the center of the ankle bone. Maintain the pressure for up to 10 minutes. Repeat every 30 minutes, as needed. **Do not use this point if you are pregnant.**

Another acupressure point that may relieve sciatic pain is found on the side of the buttock, in the depression between the top of the leg bone and the base of the hip joint.

Pain-relieving devices

TENS is highly effective at treating most nerve pain, although it does not seem to be quite as effective at treating post-herpes neuralgia. Handheld devices such as massagers/vibrators and intrasound are also effective if treatment is applied firmly enough for long enough—at least 45 minutes per session.

Reflexology

A reflexology treatment may help relieve the pain of neuralgia. For sciatica, there are specific points on the heel (see pp. 74–75).

Relaxation therapies/Yoga

Stress management techniques, such as meditation, autogenic training, and biofeedback, can be helpful.

Yoga postures that concentrate on stretching, especially those that tone the spine and back muscles, combined with yogic breathing exercises can help.

Practitioner therapies

- Cranial osteopathy
- Osteopathy and chiropractic
- Acupuncture
- Hypnotherapy
- Alexander technique

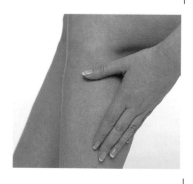

One of the acupressure points that may relieve the pain of sciatica is BL 58, on the outside of the calf muscle. It is situated on the bladder meridian.

Musculoskeletal pain

SHINGLES

An extremely painful, blistering rash around the midriff (although the neck, face, and—sometimes—the eyes can also be affected) characterizes shingles. The condition is caused by the *Herpes zoster* virus—the same virus that causes chicken pox—and results from an inflammation of the nerve roots.

Shingles most commonly occurs in older people, often as the result of a weakened immune system coinciding with a period of emotional stress.

Herbal medicine

Aloe vera can help alleviate the rash, applied either as a gel or a liquid (full strength or diluted) as required.

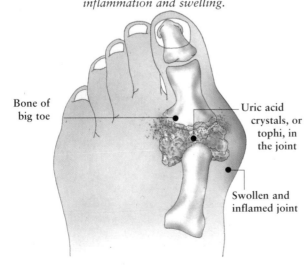

HOW GOUT DEVELOPS

If the body produces too much uric acid, or fails to excrete uric acid, excess is stored around the joints in the form of crystals. Called tophi, these deposits can be felt through the skin as small, hard lumps, and may cause inflammation and swelling.

Bone of big toe

Uric acid crystals, or tophi, in the joint

Swollen and inflamed joint

Naturopathy

A warm bath of bicarbonate of soda (1–2 cups to a bath) eases irritation. Or try an oatmeal bath: hang a 1-lb (500-g) bag of whole oats under the running tap and when the bath is half full mix in a few tablespoons of oat flour. Use the wet bag full of oats as a sponge to dab the worst affected areas.

Dietary and nutritional therapies

Eat a healthy diet and take a good-quality multivitamin and mineral supplement containing vitamins A (preferably as betacarotene), B-complex, C, and E; the mineral zinc; and the amino acid lysine.

Aromatherapy

The essential oils of geranium, sage, and thyme mixed together and rubbed, or gently dabbed, onto the affected area can help if used at the first signs of a rash. Mix three drops of each oil into 20 ml of a neutral carrier oil such as grapeseed.

Homeopathy

Use *Rhus tox* 6c for red, itching, and blistered skin; *Apis mel* if there is a burning sensation; and *Mezereum* if there is pain and itching. Apply the last two to the rash as a cold liquid or lotion.

Practitioner therapies

• Acupuncture (especially to alleviate post-herpetic neuralgia or pain following rash)

GOUT

When the body fails to process uric acid (a by-product of waste elimination), gout is the result. Crystals of uric acid build up around joints and produce swelling, redness, and pain. It commonly attacks the big toe, but the knees, elbows, and hands can also be affected.

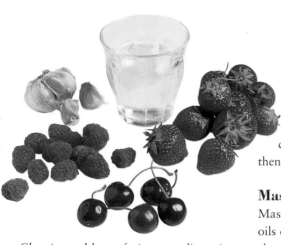

Cherries and berry fruits neutralize uric acid in the body, preventing the buildup that causes gout. Garlic boosts the immune system and may also contribute to relieving gout.

Attacks come and go, and may produce a high temperature. Constant attacks may damage the joints so recovery is harder and takes longer.

Naturopathy

A cold compress can alleviate the pain of a severe attack but longer-lasting relief may be obtained from a comfrey and calendula (marigold) poultice applied to the affected area as necessary.

A hot Epsom salts bath (add a cupful to a bath and soak for 20 minutes) also helps eliminate uric acid.

Diet and nutritional therapies

Avoid caffeine, alcohol, shellfish, sardines, organ meats, and beans; all contribute to the formation of uric acid. Drinking lots of pure, noncarbonated water and eating garlic, cherries, and berries dissolves crystals and neutralizes uric acid.

Herbal medicine

Daily infusions of burdock, nettle, wintergreen, wild carrot, sassafras, juniper, parsley, and/or willow (choose two or three) can clear the problem.

Homeopathy

Arnica and *Belladonna* can reduce the severity of an attack. Take a 6c dose every half hour for up to 10 doses (less if the pain subsides) and then 30c three times daily.

Massage and aromatherapy

Massage the affected area with essential oils of cypress, peppermint, lavender, chamomile, geranium, eucalyptus, or rosemary (2 drops in a little carrier oil). You can add 3 or 4 drops of your preferred combination to a bath.

CARPAL TUNNEL SYNDROME

Inflammation of the carpal tunnel, a tube of sinew through which the arm's nerves and tendons travel to the hand, leads to swelling that pinches the nerves and produces tingling, numbness, and pain in the index finger and thumb. The condition is common in pregnant and elderly women.

Hydrotherapy

Alternating hot and cold compresses can reduce pain and alleviate symptoms.

Diet and nutritional therapy

Supplementing a whole-food diet with a daily B-complex vitamin can be effective, especially B_6 (1 g a day) with magnesium. Results may take some weeks to show, however.

Acupressure

Pressing points on either side of the wrist firmly for two minutes can relieve pain. One point is on the underside of the wrist and the other is on the wrist's top center, where the hand joins the arm. ▶

Find out more	
Aromatherapy	36
Acupressure	38
Acupuncture	68

Proprietary wristbands—often marketed as preventing seasickness—apply pressure to the points on either side of the wrist. In this way they may relieve the pain caused by carpal tunnel syndrome.

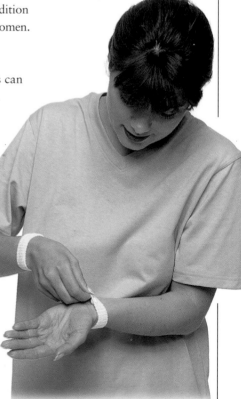

Musculoskeletal pain

NECK ACHE

An ache in the neck can be caused by any number of factors, from emotional stress, simply sitting or lying too long in one position, to more serious problems such as infection and injury.

Untreated, neck ache can result in a chronic condition needing patience and care to correct. You may also develop other symptoms such as headaches, dizziness, aching eyes, blurred vision, and jaw ache. A mild ache in the neck can be helped by simply massaging the area with your hand until the ache goes. A more severe ache, such as crick or stiff neck, where the head is stuck at an uncomfortable angle and is painful to move, needs more careful treatment.

A massage to the neck, shoulders, and upper back can be an effective cure for neck ache, as well as relieving general tension.

Warning: A stiff neck for no obvious reason, with a worsening headache, high temperature, and sensitivity to light, is one of the first symptoms of meningitis, an extremely dangerous infection of the meninges, the protective membranes that envelop the brain and spinal cord and contain the cerebrospinal fluid. Immediate medical help should be sought if these symptoms are experienced.

Massage and aromatherapy

Stroke down the side of the neck and across the shoulders a few times, keeping the muscles relaxed and your hands molded to the contours of your body. Next, knead the muscles and tissues of the neck and shoulders with the palms and fingers of one hand. Start gently and feel for knots or areas that are hard and tender, working them until the hardness goes. Hold any tender areas in the neck or shoulders firmly and stretch the warmed muscles by slowly circling your shoulders or head, effectively getting them to massage themselves.

Using a few drops of the essential oils of marjoram and/or rosemary diluted in a carrier oil adds to the benefit. Getting a friend or partner to massage your neck and shoulders is even more effective—but be careful to avoid the throat area.

Reflexology

Apply pressure to the areas on both feet where the big toes join the sole—they are said to correspond to the neck. For severe neck ache, consult a qualified reflexologist.

Pain-relieving devices

TENS (transcutaneous nerve stimulation) can provide very effective pain relief, as can other devices that encourage blood into the area, such as intrasound and massagers (see pp. 59 and 83). TENS should not be applied near the throat.

Practitioner therapies

• Physiotherapy

• Movement therapies such as yoga, t'ai chi, Alexander technique, the Feldenkrais method, Rolfing, and Hellerwork

WHIPLASH

Pain in the neck, and sometimes also the back, can be caused by the head being jolted severely backward. It is common as a result of car accidents, especially when there are no headrests. The pain is the result of the muscles, tendons, and ligaments in the neck being strained and attempting to heal. Symptoms can also include headaches, disturbed vision, fatigue, pins and needles, anxiety, and depression. Whiplash may become apparent immediately after a jolt, or it may develop later.

Naturopathy

For mild cases, alternating hot and cold compresses can bring immediate relief, as can a very gentle massage to encourage blood to the area.

Homeopathy

Arnica tincture or ointment rubbed gently into the affected area helps to ease bruising, provided it is applied within an hour of the accident or jolt. *Arnica* 30c, in pill form, can also be taken (one every 5 minutes) for the first 30 minutes after the incident, followed by *hypericum* 6c every 4 hours, for up to 3 days.

Pain-relieving devices

As for neck ache.

Nutritional therapy

To relieve stiffness, take calcium pantothenate. To help tissue repair, take a good multivitamin and mineral supplement that also contains amino acids. Daily doses of vitamin C (3–5 g), calcium (1 g), and magnesium (500 mg) help acute pain. Fish oil capsules (EPA) with gammalinoleic acid (GLA) may help. The freshwater alga spirulina, available in powder form from retail health outlets, is also recommended.

Relaxation therapies

You should encourage relaxation of the neck muscles by avoiding stress, a cause of muscular tension. Therapies such as meditation, visualization, biofeedback, self-hypnosis, and affirmations can all help promote mental and emotional relaxation (see pp. 46–51).

Practitioner therapies

• Acupuncture

• Osteopathy and chiropractic

• Cranial osteopathy

TORTICOLLIS (WRY NECK)

Spasm of the muscles on either side of the neck result in torticolli or wry neck. It can be chronic as well as acute. In its chronic state, it is more often a genetic problem, rather than one caused by injury or illness; acute torticollis can be caused by an inflamed gland or rheumatism in the area.

Congenital wry neck is difficult to correct after childhood without surgery, but the same approaches that are helpful for neck pain can alleviate any discomfort from short-term spasm. ▶

Musculoskeletal pain

BACK PAIN

Back ache or pain is one of the most common types of pain. More working days are lost in the Western world through back problems, all of which are painful to varying degrees, than any other illness except the flu. The back is a complex structure of bones—the vertebrae—covered with interconnecting muscles and tissues, responsible for holding us upright. This puts the back under constant strain, and is the reason why back problems are difficult to treat.

Although pain can occur anywhere in the back, the majority of back pain occurs in the lower back, where it is better known as lumbago. Conventional treatments are drugs such as muscle relaxants, anti-inflammatories, steroids, antidepressants, and tranquilizers—all of which can have side effects.

The majority (about 90 percent) of episodes of back pain settle within six weeks. Occasionally pain may become chronic and physical therapy, osteopathy, and sometimes surgery may be required.

ACUTE BACK PAIN TREATMENT

No more than 24 hours bed rest is recommended. Continue to work if possible and get some exercise. See your doctor if you have a history of cancer, if you have a fever, have suffered a blow, or if there is any disturbance of sensation, bladder, or bowel function.

Naturopathy

Cold and hot compresses can help ease the pain. With an ice pack and a covered hot-water bottle, apply hot and cold compresses alternately. Apply the ice pack for 10 minutes and the hot pack for 5 minutes, alternating for as long and as often as the treatment helps.

Pain-relieving devices

TENS machines can provide very effective pain relief, as can devices that encourage blood into the area, such as intrasound and vibrating massagers (see pp. 59 and 83). If using massagers, high-frequency ones, applied for at least 45 minutes, tend to give the best results.

Massage and aromatherapy

Ask a friend or partner to massage your whole back carefully, concentrating on "hot" spots or areas of pain, but not applying pressure to the spine itself.

A mixture of 12 drops of ginger, 5 drops of juniper, and 8 drops of either rosemary or lavender oil (rosemary is stimulating and lavender calming) added to a carrier oil will make the massage more effective. Other oils beneficial for acute pain are black pepper, cypress, birch, and eucalyptus. For general muscle ache, try marjoram, chamomile, or clary sage.

Herbal medicine

Bromelain (pineapple extract) is a powerful anti-inflammatory (take 2–3 g daily at first, then 1–2 g as the pain eases). Other anti-inflammatories, effective when drunk as teas, are valerian, St. John's wort, and Jamaican dogwood.

Natural aspirin tablets made from willow bark and meadowsweet can help relieve pain. Ginger, cayenne, horseradish, lobelia, and cramp bark rubbed into the painful area aid recovery by stimulating local blood flow.

Homeopathy

If the pain or ache is from a strain or injury, *Arnica* tincture or ointment rubbed gently into the affected area will help ease any bruising if it is applied within an hour of the incident.

Taking *Arnica* 6c every half hour for up to 3 hours, then every 4 hours for up to 5 days is effective. *Rhus tox* 3c is good for muscular strain and *Ruta* 3c for bruised bones and tendons.

Practitioner therapies
- Acupuncture
- Chiropractic and osteopathy
- Cranial osteopathy/craniosacral therapy
- Physiotherapy
- Hypnotherapy/hypnosis
- Massage

CHRONIC BACK PAIN TREATMENT
Hydrotherapy
Swimming combined with a sauna or steam bathing (hydrotherapy) is excellent for relieving back pain.

Exercise
Gentle exercise is widely accepted as being much better for back problems than total rest, although it is important not to overexert yourself during the healing process. Cycling can be beneficial, as can swimming because in both your body weight is supported. Walking and jogging are also effective (but wear suitable shoes for walking and appropriate trainers for jogging). Once you are on the road to recovery, yoga or t'ai chi may be beneficial. It is a good idea to have a few lessons from a trained teacher so that you do the movements correctly from the start and do not learn bad habits.

Dietary and nutritional therapies
Eating a healthy and nutritious diet and avoiding unhealthy foods are as important for back pain as they are for any other painful condition. Eat plenty of fresh fruit and vegetables, and try to cut down on—or even eliminate—animal fats, sugar, salt, alcohol, tea, and coffee. Supplements of fish oils (EPA) combined with evening primrose/starflower oils (GLA) are recommended. A good multivitamin and mineral preparation with vitamin C, calcium, magnesium, and manganese will also help.

Aromatherapy
Regular hot (but not uncomfortably hot) baths containing a few drops each of chamomile, lavender, juniper, eucalyptus, and rosemary oils help relieve pain. ▶

Find out more	
Hydrotherapy	62
Drug therapy	80
Physiotherapy	82

The constant demands placed on the spine and muscles of the back mean that back problems affect more people than almost any other condition. Although painful, most back problems resolve themselves with time and gentle exercise.

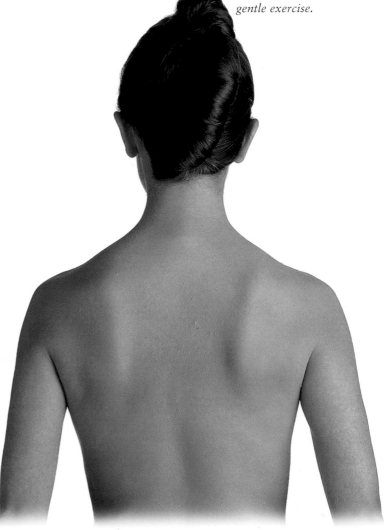

Musculoskeletal pain

Alexander technique

The Alexander technique teaches correct postural habits and is particularly effective for neck and back pain if practiced regularly.

Reflexology

Gently apply pressure with your thumb to one of the reflexology points for the back. Hold for 1 minute. The area corresponding to the spine runs along the inner edge of both feet, from the toe to the heel. Press the base of the big toe for upper back pain; below the ball of the foot for middle back pain; and in the arch for lower pain back. Consider consulting a trained reflexologist if pain persists.

A reflexology treatment for lower back pain would include pressure applied to the instep.

Relaxation therapies

These encourage relaxation of the back muscles by avoiding stress—a common cause of muscular tension. Therapies such as meditation, visualization, biofeedback, self-hypnosis, and affirmations can all help promote mental and emotional relaxation (see pp. 46–51).

Practitioner therapies

- Acupuncture
- Chiropractic
- Massage
- Osteopathy
- Cranial osteopathy/craniosacral therapy
- Physiotherapy
- Hellerwork
- Rolfing
- Feldenkrais method
- Hypnotherapy/hypnosis
- Healing/therapeutic touch

SLIPPED DISK

Between each vertebra in the spine is a flat disk of springy cartilage that acts as a shock absorber. This can sometimes squeeze or slip out of place, for example as the result of an awkward movement. Magnetic resonance imaging scans show that about one third of the population have slipped disks, most of which cause no problems. Most slipped disks resolve themselves with time. However, if the disk presses on a nerve it can cause pain down the leg (known as sciatica). Acute trauma may produce a tear in the disk and some disk material may squeeze out to produce pressure and inflammation of a nerve.

The pain caused by a slipped disk is sudden, severe, and often accompanied by spasm of the back muscles, pins and needles, and numbness in one or both legs or feet. If this happens seek the help of a qualified osteopath, chiropractor, or doctor as soon as possible. Manipulation of the spine can relieve pressure on the nerve and thus eliminate the pain. Severe

---

SLIPPED DISK

Most slipped disks result from the way the disks and spine are formed, although twisting movements can damage the casing of an intervertebral disk, causing the disk to bulge out.

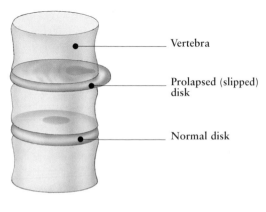

Vertebra

Prolapsed (slipped) disk

Normal disk

pain may require surgical intervention; surgery may also be necessary if bladder or bowel function is affected.

Electronic devices

A TENS device can provide immediate pain relief (see p. 83).

Hydrotherapy

Apply alternate hot and cold compresses to the area. Heat may help, so hold a covered hot-water bottle to your back.

Homeopathy

Try *Arnica* 6c every half hour for up to three hours and then once every 4 hours for up to 5 days.

Practitioner therapies

- Acupuncture
- Chiropractic
- Osteopathy
- Physiotherapy

KYPHOSIS

The condition in which the thoracic (upper) spine has an abnormally increased convexity in the curvature when viewed from the side is known as kyphosis. The most common postural problem, this results in a hunchback appearance. It is often seen in those who spend most of their time sitting. It may also result from osteoporosis.

Treatment should concentrate on regular exercises that promote posture correction and deep breathing. It is also important to make sure that work surfaces are at the correct height and to learn to relax.

LORDOSIS

Sitting too much or standing for too long with the knees locked backward may cause lordosis, an abnormally increased concavity in the curvature of the lumbar (lower) spine, when viewed from the side. It may be exacerbated by tightness of the back muscles. ▶

The Feldenkrais method is said to be effective in treating back pain. Gentle massage helps you tune in to your body and become aware of where you are holding tension.

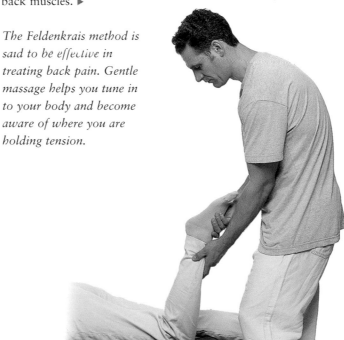

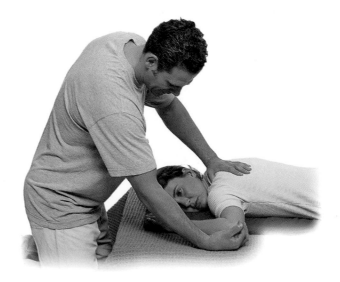

Musculoskeletal pain

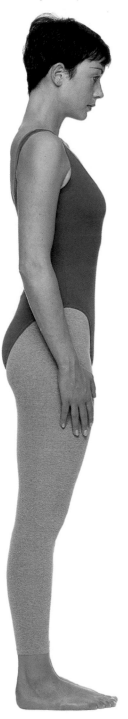

To counter lordosis, stand on the balls of your feet and pull in your chin.

To correct lordosis, stand tall, but relax your knees. Stand with your pelvis tilted slightly forward and stomach muscles gently pulled in. Tuck your chin in to lengthen the back of your neck and help reduce the common "poked forward" look. Exercises to strengthen stomach muscles will also help.

SCOLIOSIS

Scoliosis is a curvature of the spine to one side, with twisting. It is common in varying degrees and the cause is often unknown. It occurs as a congenital defect or may be due to muscle spasm on one side of the spine, or muscle paralysis. Occasionally it is postural. Scoliosis can interfere with lung function and produce compression of the nerves as they leave the spine.

In severe cases a lift fitted into a shoe will help. Regularly stretching the muscles of the hips and trunk helps straighten the spine. Cranial osteopathy can also help. Severe cases require specialist treatment.

Posture training

To help learn new posture habits, seek professional help from a specialist in one of the following therapies:
• Osteopathy and chiropractic
• Physiotherapy
• Massage therapy
• Yoga
• T'ai chi
• Alexander technique
• Feldenkrais method
• Rolfing
• Hellerwork

CRAMPS

Cramps are a sudden muscle spasm that occur frequently after strenuous exercise, at night, and during pregnancy. Cramps occur in response to nerve stimuli, but the exact cause of the condition is unknown. Cramps are common and usually last no more than a few minutes.

Naturopathy

Press hard into the center of the painful area with the thumbs and try to stretch the muscle at the same time. Stretching affects nerve activity in the area, leading to a relaxation of the muscle, easing the cramp. As soon as possible, apply a towel soaked in hot water and wrung out. Repeat the application 4 or 5 times every 5 minutes and then gently work the muscle by rubbing, stretching, and kneading it.

Herbal medicine

Take kelp or ginkgo biloba in tablet or capsule form, or cramp bark as a tea.

Homeopathy

The remedy *Cuprum metallicum* 3c can help prevent and alleviate attacks.

Dietary and nutritional therapies

Eating plenty of dark green leafy vegetables, shellfish, nuts, and seeds can help prevent attacks, particularly if you are prone to cramps. Alternatively, supplement your diet with evening primrose or starflower oils (1 g a day), vitamins C (3 g) and E (250–400 iu), and calcium and magnesium.

OTHER MUSCULOSKELETAL PROBLEMS

Pain and stiffness in the muscles is known as fibrositis, or fibromyalgia. Although the cause of fibromyalgia is still unknown, it may be due to poor posture, may occur following an infection or after unaccustomed exercise.

Tendinitis (inflammation of tendons) is caused by repetitive use or by injury. Inflammation of the tendons is responsible for such conditions as repetitive strain injury (RSI) and tennis elbow. Tenosynovitis is an inflammation of the tendon and its synovial sheath. It may be caused by overuse or repetitive action, or —occasionally—by bacterial infection.

Bursitis is an inflammation of the bursa, the soft tissues covering joints that allow them to move. It usually results from pressure or friction, but is occasionally caused by bacterial infection. Inflammation of the bursa is responsible for such conditions as frozen shoulder and housemaid's knee.

These conditions are always painful, incapacitating, and sometimes chronic. Time and gentle exercise can often cure acute occurrences. Rest is not usually helpful since it deconditions the muscles.

Naturopathy

Apply cold compresses at the first sign of inflammation as often as it helps. If the inflammation is severe, apply regular ice packs. Once improvement starts, change to alternating hot and cold compresses and begin gentle exercise to keep the joints mobile.

Dietary and nutritional therapies

Fresh fruit and vegetables, particularly celery, promote recovery. Supplement with a range of nutrients, especially essential fatty

Nutritional supplements including evening primrose oil can be effective for cramps.

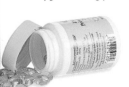

acids (EPA and GLA), vitamins A, C, E, and B-complex, magnesium and calcium, and the enzymes bromelain and papain. Avoid tea, coffee, alcohol, sugar, and acid-containing fruits.

Herbal medicine

Hot teas of valerian, bogbean, goldenseal, willow, and primula promote recovery, and chamomile with hops or passionflower at night aids relaxation and sleep.

Hot herbal poultices can also be effective, particularly using comfrey, marsh mallow, slippery elm, and flaxseed.

Homeopathy

Try *Arnica* 6c or apis 6c every 2 hours for acute inflammation, *Rhus tox* 6c or *Bryonia* 6c twice daily for 2 weeks for recurrent attacks. See a qualified therapist for an individual prescription.

Massage and aromatherapy

Massage with essential oils of lavender, sandalwood, juniper, eucalyptus, thyme, and/or rosemary (5 drops diluted in a little carrier oil). Knead rather than smooth the affected areas.

Hot baths with rosemary and/or pine oils added (10 drops) are beneficial.

Acupressure

For a frozen shoulder, applying pressure upward to either end of the upper arm bone (humerus) can help. Hold for up to 3 minutes each time. Repeat daily.

Practitioner therapies

- Acupuncture
- Hypnotherapy
- Chinese herbal medicine
- Osteopathy or chiropractic

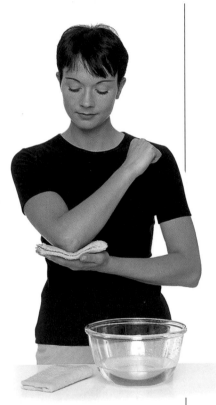

Applying a cold compress can often relieve the pain of tennis elbow.

Musculoskeletal pain

ARTHRITIS

There are many different types—more than 100 varieties have been identified—of arthritis, a degenerative joint disease. It is one of the most common and most severe forms of pain, affecting an estimated 10 percent of the population. The two main types are osteoarthritis and rheumatoid arthritis. Nonconventional therapies now have such a good record in the treatment of both forms—for prevention and cure—that they are the treatments of choice of many doctors over conventional drug therapy.

OSTEOARTHRITIS

This condition is caused by the gradual wearing down of the protective cartilage between the joints and consequent damage to the bones themselves, leading to pain, reduced movement, and deformity of the joint. It is the most common form of arthritis and is experienced mainly in the hips, knees, and hands. It affects men and women equally.

RHEUMATOID ARTHRITIS

Rheumatoid arthritis affects all the body's tissues, especially the joints, causing inflammation. It usually begins in the hands and feet and spreads to the rest of the body. It is an autoimmune disease, which means that the body turns against itself and attacks its own tissues.

Diet, lifestyle, stress, and genetic predisposition are widely regarded as the main causes. Women are 3–4 times more likely to suffer than men, especially between the ages of 20 and 40. Apart from swelling, stiffness, and pain in the affected joints, producing a characteristically red and shiny skin, sufferers may experience fatigue, loss of appetite, and often a slight temperature.

An extract from the New Zealand green-lipped mussel has been recommended as a supplement for rheumatoid arthritis.

Naturopathy

For pain relief, both hot and cold compresses are effective. Bathing can also help. Choose from seawater, seaweed (bladderwrack), or Epsom salts (3–4 tablespoons in a hot bath).

Juice fasts of freshly pressed fruits and vegetables have been successful in treating arthritis. A combination of celery, carrot, beet, potato, white cabbage, and cucumber is recommended.

Gentle daily exercise is important for both forms of arthritis. Swimming is excellent (together with a sauna or steam bath), as is gentle walking. Wearing a copper bracelet or elastic supports impregnated with copper may help.

Dietary and nutritional therapies

Reduce consumption of animal fats, tea, coffee, and alcohol, and drink plenty of clean, pure water every day—at least 6–8 glasses.

Eat lots of fresh fruit and vegetables but avoid acid-producing foods, such as red meat, tomatoes, and citrus fruit. An extract of the New Zealand green-lipped mussel (available as a capsule from health-food stores) and drinking cider vinegar mixed with honey three times a day with meals is said to be beneficial.

Recommended daily food supplements include high doses of fish oils balanced with omega-3 oils. Vitamins A, C, E, and B-complex; the minerals zinc, iron, magnesium, manganese, copper, molybdenum, selenium, and silica; the enzyme superoxide dismutase; and the amino acid complex glutathione are all said to help relieve arthritis. All these supplements are normally included in a good-quality multivitamin and mineral tablet but fish oils must be taken separately as liquid or capsules.

Herbal medicine

Herbs to reduce inflammation include capsaicin (cayenne) cream, celery seeds, yucca, bogbean, devil's claw, black cohosh, wild yam, willow bark, and feverfew. Seek the help of a trained herbalist for an individual prescription.

Homeopathy

Ruta graveolens cream rubbed into the affected area helps. Rhus tox, *Ruta grav, arnica*, and *Bryonia* can be taken as pills. Refer to a qualified therapist.

Massage and aromatherapy

Massage with 2 or 3 drops of lavender and/or chamomile essential oils combined in a little carrier oil. Cypress, eucalyptus, and rosemary, either massaged in, or added to a bath, can help. ▶

Find out more

Musculoskeletal system	*18*
Nutritional therapy	*33*
Exercise	*52*

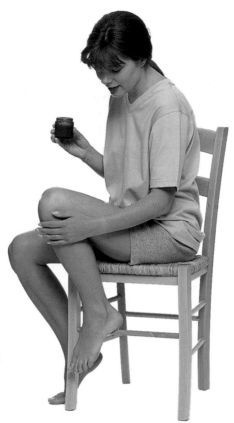

A cream based on the homeopathic remedy Ruta graveolens *can be applied directly to painful joints.*

ESSENTIAL FATTY ACIDS

OMEGA-3 CHEMICAL NAME Alphalinoleic acid

KEY INGREDIENTS	BEST SUPPLEMENT SOURCES	BEST FOOD SOURCES
Eicosapentaenoic acid (EPA)	Marine or fish oils	Oily fish (tuna, mackerel, herring)
Gammalinoleic acid (GLA)	Blackcurrant seed oil	Dark green leafy vegetables
	Flaxseed (linseed) oil	Sunflower seeds
	Evening primrose oil	Safflower and sesame seeds
	Starflower (borage) oil	Pumpkin seeds, oats, wheat, rice
		Peas and beans

OMEGA-6 CHEMICAL NAME Linoleic acid

KEY INGREDIENTS	BEST SUPPLEMENT SOURCES	BEST FOOD SOURCES
Linoleic acid	Flaxseed (linseed) oil	Sunflower and sesame seeds
	Blackcurrant seed oil	Extra virgin olive oil

It is important to take omega-3 and omega-6 EFAs in combination and most experts now agree that the right ratio is two omega-3s to one omega-6. This combination is now widely available in a single capsule from pharmacies and health-food stores.

Musculoskeletal pain

Movement therapies

Yoga and t'ai chi exercise routines are excellent for all types of arthritis because they are gentle and encourage the right mental and emotional approach to dealing with pain. Dance movement offers a less structured, more free-flowing alternative. Initially, instruction is required from a qualified practitioner.

Acupressure

Practice every morning and evening while symptoms last, keeping up the pressure for about two minutes each time.
• For knee pain: Press a point on the front of the leg, four fingers' width below the bottom of the kneecap and about a finger's width to the outside of the shin bone.
• For hip pain: Press in firmly at the sides of the hips in the hollow where the leg joins the pelvis.
• For hand pain: Press in toward the forefinger at the end of the webs of skin between forefinger and thumb.

Reflexology

Manipulating the whole foot—sole, sides, and top—is recommended since this will cover the many reflex points involved in arthritis, particularly systemic (whole-body) rheumatoid arthritis (see pp. 74–75).

Electronic devices

TENS can help relieve pain effectively in both the high- and low-frequency ranges. Experimentation is needed to find what works for you. Handheld devices such as massagers/vibrators and intrasound are also effective if used firmly enough for long enough (at least 45 minutes).

Relaxation therapies

Visualization, meditation, and biofeedback have a good record of helping with arthritic pain but initial instruction is necessary from a good practitioner (see pp. 46–51).

Practitioner therapies

• Acupuncture for pain relief
• Chinese herbal medicine
• Cranial osteopathy (especially for rheumatoid arthritis)
• Osteopathy or chiropractic for the alleviation of chronic but not acute conditions
• Psychotherapy and counseling
• Hypnotherapy

Pain in the joints may be relieved using acupressure techniques. Illustrated below (left to right) are points for the hand, hip, and knee.

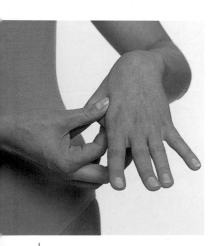
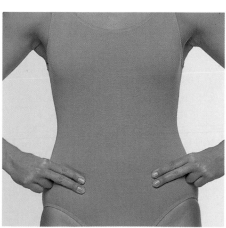
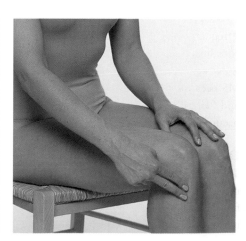

MULTIPLE SCLEROSIS

Known as MS for short, multiple sclerosis is a disease of the central nervous system caused by inflammation of, and subsequent damage to, the myelin sheath, the fatty coating surrounding the nerve fibers. This leads to a wide variety of symptoms as a result of interference with nerve signals to the brain, including tingling or pins and needles in the limbs, blurred vision, numbness, difficulty walking, loss of coordination, fatigue, depression, and various muscular aches and pains.

MS is a degenerative and at present incurable condition and, as yet, its causes are unknown. The symptoms are so complex that it is more usefully seen as a collection of variable symptoms rather than a single disease. For reasons still unclear, it is more common in colder climates and affects women more than men. Conventional medicine can treat some of its symptoms, but has little to offer to treat the condition itself.

Depending on the severity of symptoms and how long-standing the problem is, the condition can be helped considerably—and sometimes arrested—by a variety of non-drug therapies.

Physical therapies

A regular routine of muscle-stretching, coordination, and strengthening exercises is extremely beneficial for anyone with MS because it helps to retain mobility and flexibility and overcome pains that occur from lack of use.

Dietary and nutritional therapies

There is evidence that symptoms can be made worse by eating too much animal fat, dairy products, sugar, and salt. Also, it appears that people with MS lack, or do not adequately metabolize, certain important nutrients, particularly vitamin B_{12}. Eating a whole-food diet with lots of fresh fruit and vegetables, brown rice, and whole grains will help. The following food supplements can be particularly helpful for MS.
- Essential fatty acids: polyunsaturated omega-3 and omega-6, taken as capsules
- Vitamins and minerals: vitamin A (preferably as betacarotene); the B-vitamins, especially B_1, B_2, B_3, B_6, B_{12}, biotin; vitamin C; vitamin E; zinc, magnesium, manganese, molybdenum, selenium, and vanadium

Seek advice on dosage from a qualified nutritional therapist because individual needs will vary depending on symptoms.

Massage and aromatherapy

Massaging aching and painful muscles and limbs with essential oils is as useful in MS as in any other condition. The list of oils that can be used is long, so help is best sought from a qualified clinical aromatherapist. Once you have received advice on the right oil or combination of oils for individual symptoms, you can apply the same oils at home.

Examples of useful massage oils are chamomile for bladder and bowels; black pepper, juniper, and rosemary for muscle tone; clary sage and jasmine to ease tension; and basil, rosemary, nutmeg, thyme, geranium, and marjoram for fatigue.

Reflexology

Manipulating the feet can help many of the symptoms of MS, including bladder and bowel problems, fatigue, depression, and sexual problems. See a qualified therapist first, since techniques vary according to individual symptoms.

Digestive and urinary pain

Many digestive and urinary problems have relatively minor causes, but they can cause great pain. There is a wide range of self-help therapies, but bear in mind that some conditions (appendicitis, for example) require urgent medical attention.

NAUSEA

Feeling sick, or nauseated, may result from eating and drinking too much or unwisely, food poisoning, motion (travel) sickness, pregnancy, and migraines. It is normally accompanied by the urge to vomit. Certain illnesses and drug treatments may also cause nausea.

Dietary therapy

Vomiting is a natural response to a stomach upset and should not be suppressed. After vomiting, rinse your mouth with water. Eat clear soups and "neutral" foods such as rice, dry toast, boiled vegetables, and pears for 24 hours to allow the system to recover.

Clear soup, boiled vegetables, and pears are among the light foods that help recovery after an attack of vomiting.

Warning: Persistent vomiting may be a sign of serious illness; consult your doctor. Vomiting blood should always be investigated by a medical practitioner.

Herbal medicine

Ginger, taken as a tea, as capsules (swallow two half an hour before traveling), or by chewing the raw root, is effective for all forms of sickness and nausea, especially those caused by motion (car, air, and sea sickness). To make a tea, cut the root into pieces, simmer for about 15 minutes and drink. Ginger is particularly effective if drunk with peppermint tea. Eating crystallized ginger during a journey may help to relieve motion sickness. Teas of Roman chamomile and black horehound reduce nausea and vomiting. These herbs should not be taken during pregnancy.

Acupressure

Press a point on the wrist in line with the middle finger, three fingers' width from the inner wrist crease. A point in the middle of the stomach, between the breastbone and the navel, can have a similar effect. Press firmly for several seconds. Elasticated bands with a sewn-in pressure stud that can be worn on the wrist during a journey to help keep sickness at bay ("seabands") are available from many pharmacists and health stores.

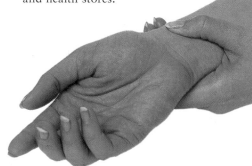

The acupressure point known as Pericardium 6 is effective for controlling nausea and vomiting.

Homeopathy

The following homeopathic remedies (all 6c) are recommended: *Nux vomica* and *Cocculus* for general vomiting and nausea; *Sepia* for nausea brought on by the smell of food; *Pulsatilla*, *Ipecacuanha*, and *Arsenicum alb* for motion sickness and vomiting after eating; *Tabacum* if the symptoms include sweating and giddiness; and *Borax* if there is accompanying anxiety.

Aromatherapy

Add four drops of essential oil of peppermint to a neutral carrier oil such as grapeseed and rub onto the chest. Alternatively, put the drops onto a tissue or handkerchief and breathe in the vapor.

Practitioner therapies

- Acupuncture
- Chinese herbal medicine

INDIGESTION

Indigestion or dyspepsia (heartburn) is characterized by a burning pain in the center of the chest. The cause is acid in the stomach backing up into the gullet, usually from eating and drinking too much, too quickly. Symptoms are similar to those for an ulcer, hiatal hernia, or heart attack so they must taken seriously, even though indigestion is the most likely cause of chest pain.

Dietary and nutritional therapies

For quick relief, sip cider vinegar or lemon juice in hot water and apply a hot-water bottle to the area. If the indigestion is severe, it is best to follow this with a 12-hour fast, drinking only herb teas (see Herbal medicines, right) or crushed apple or carrot juice. Taking a tablespoon of whey concentrate (milk serum) regularly with meals, is said to be the best regulator of stomach acids in the long term, but prevention is the main aim.

Always eat in as relaxed a manner as possible and try not to rush meals. Eat little and often, rather than big meals,

infrequently. A varied diet, combining lots of fresh fruit and vegetables with carbohydrates (such as pasta) and proteins (such as fish) will also help. Keep your fat intake to a minimum. Taking regular acidophilus and pectin supplements can also help prevent indigestion.

Herbal medicine

Meadowsweet, coriander, and slippery elm tablets (or powders) taken with warm water aid indigestion pain, as do teas of ginger, peppermint, chamomile, parsley, fennel, lemon balm, raspberry leaf, and cinnamon. Ginger and parsley eaten raw work as well.

Reflexology

Apply pressure across the whole of the middle of the sole of each foot—the area corresponding to the digestive and elimination organs. Press firmly on any points of tenderness until they disperse (see pp. 74–75).

Practitioner therapies

- Acupuncture
- Chinese herbal medicine ▶

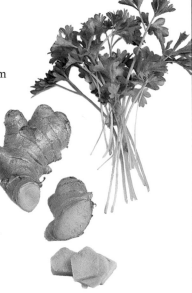

Eating raw ginger or parsley can control acidity and so relieve indigestion.

TREATMENT FOR HANGOVERS

The best way to avoid a hangover is not to indulge in excessive amounts of alcohol. To help prevent a hangover, drink at least one glass of milk before drinking large amounts of alcohol. Before going to bed, drink as much water as possible. This will prevent the dehydration that causes a headache. The next day drink an infusion of peppermint, chamomile, nettle, or yarrow. Large amounts of honey (12 tsp), full strength or in warm water, may help. Morning-after cures include a raw egg in Worcestershire sauce or cider vinegar; the homeopathic remedy Nux vomica 6c; *and the herbal extract spirulina.*

Digestive and urinary pain

STOMACHACHE

One of the most common pains, stomachache is most often the result of eating the wrong foods or too much food. It may be accompanied by nausea, but it does not usually last long. Anxiety and tension are also causes.

Warning: Severe stomach pain that is prolonged or recurs for no obvious reason should be reported to a doctor as soon as possible.

Applying a hot water bottle can be comforting and is a simple way to relieve a stomachache.

Dietary and nutritional therapies

A hot water bottle on the stomach can bring immediate relief. For pain from overeating and drinking, or eating the wrong food,

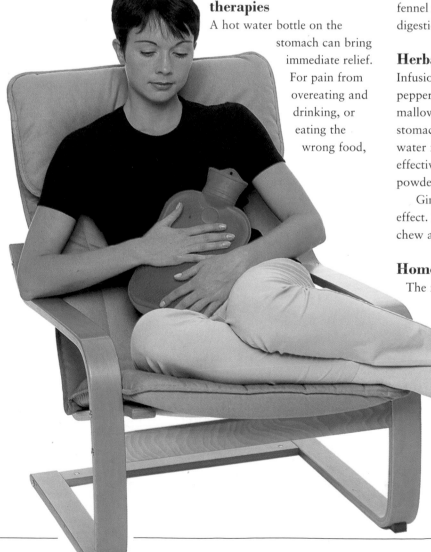

a minifast—not eating for 12 hours—is most effective. It is important to drink plenty of water for the duration of a fast and not to drink coffee, tea, or alcohol.

For prevention of a stomachache, eat little and often instead of a lot all at once, and eat healthily (whole foods, and fresh fruit and vegetables). You should try reducing the intake of fatty foods as much as possible. Not exercising too soon after eating (wait at least 30 minutes and preferably a full hour) and wearing loose clothing can also help.

Apple juice with ginger, mint, and fennel is said to be effective. It can aid digestion and also dispel gas.

Herbal medicine

Infusions (teas) of chamomile, peppermint, lemon balm, or marsh mallow are soothing and relaxing on the stomach. Infuse the dried herbs in boiling water for 5 minutes. Slippery elm is also effective, taken as either a tablet or powder dissolved in hot water.

Ginger is also said to have a calming effect. It can be taken as a tea, or you can chew a thin slice of raw fresh ginger.

Homeopathy

The remedies *Arsenicum alb* 6c and *Bryonia* 6c or *Nux vomica* 6c or 30c are commonly prescribed. Take 1 tablet every hour for 3 hours, as needed.

Acupressure

Pressing a point on the cheek either side of and below the nose directly underneath the eyes can relieve a stomachache that is caused by stress.

Another point is on the leg, four fingers' width below the kneecap on the outside of the shinbone. This point is useful for all digestive problems.

For a general tonic, lie flat on a firm surface and press down vertically in two parallel lines from the breastbone to about halfway to the navel.

Relaxation therapies

A standard progressive muscle relaxation exercise (see pp. 46–47) followed by visualization, biofeedback, and meditation can help recurring stomachache brought on by tension and anxiety.

Movement therapies

A variety of yoga and t'ai chi routines can help pain caused by both physical and psychological causes. The yoga posture called the pose of tranquillity, for example, is said to be particularly effective for a stomachache.

Exercise

You will not want to exercise while you are experiencing pain, but regular exercise is a useful preventive measure because it stimulates digestion.

Practitioner therapies

• Acupuncture
• Chinese herbal medicine

Popular herbal teas for relieving stomach pains, especially if they are of a digestive origin, include peppermint and chamomile.

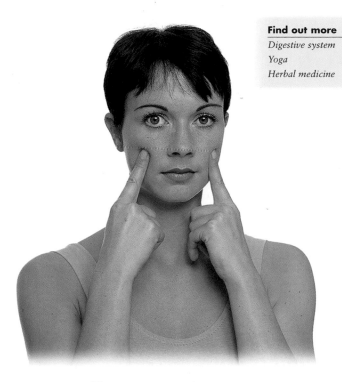

Find out more	
Digestive system	20
Yoga	40
Herbal medicine	60

The acupressure point directly below the pupils of the eyes and level with the base of the nose can help ease a stomachache associated with stress.

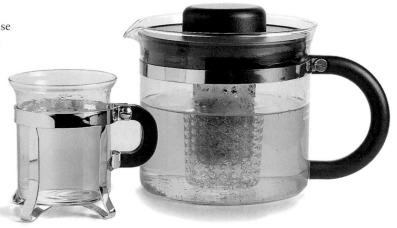

Digestive and urinary pain

CONSTIPATION

Regular bowel movements are vital for full bodily health, but "regular" can vary for each person. Anything between 3 bowel movements a day to 1 every 3 days is regarded as normal.

Constipation occurs when there is a change in the normal pattern, and stools are so hard they are uncomfortable to pass. It is most often caused by a poor diet and lack of exercise, coupled with stress.

Constipation allows toxins to seep into the blood stream, from where they spread through the body and cause such symptoms as headache and fatigue, joint and muscle pain, and allergic reactions.

Warning: A change in bowel habit may be an early warning sign of cancer of the bowel. Seek medical advice.

Naturopathy

To help cure constipation, eat natural laxatives such as prunes, fresh fruit and vegetables, and bran.

A covered hot water bottle placed on the abdomen can help, and flaxseed (linseed) oil taken with psyllium husks can clean out a sluggish colon. Regular exercise is essential and relaxation exercises if anxiety is a factor. In severe cases, it may be worth considering colonic irrigation.

Dietary and nutritional therapies

Prunes and prune juice are an excellent natural laxative, but only in the short term. Never take laxatives long term. The best approach is to increase fiber intake (bran, grains, fresh fruit, raw vegetables, and brown rice) and avoid refined foods, especially sugar and white flour. Drink at least 6–8 glasses daily of water, preferably filtered. A glass of juice with 1 tsp of wheat germ stirred into it provides a good source of fiber. Make sure your diet contains potassium (in most good multivitamin tablets). Juices of carrot or celery with garlic and onion can help.

Herbal medicine

Senna pods and cascara bark made into teas are powerful laxatives, but can cause stomach pain in the process. Chamomile, hops, and fennel help counteract this, but a gentler alternative is flaxseed (linseed) oil (a tablespoon morning and evening) or dandelion. Eat the leaves or root with a salad or make a tea and drink three times daily. Or try cape aloes and slippery elm.

Massage and aromatherapy

Massage a blend of oils of black pepper (5 drops), marjoram, and rosemary (10 drops each) into the abdomen and lower back.

Reflexology

Manipulating the whole of the middle area of the sole of the foot (corresponding to the main digestive organs) may help.

DIARRHEA

The opposite of constipation, diarrhea is waste matter that is too liquid—usually as

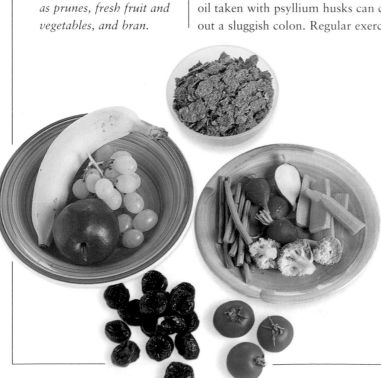

COLONIC IRRIGATION

Some naturopaths advocate washing out the whole of the large intestine, in a process called colonic irrigation. Also known as colonic hydrotherapy, this is an internal bath administered by a therapist with special equipment.

The procedure involves inserting a small hoselike device with two tubes into the rectum. One of the tubes pumps water in and the other draws it out again. Impacted feces that may be blocking the system are said to be flushed out. Irrigation is a more drastic procedure than an enema, which can be self-administered, and is not without risks and dangers. Practitioners need to be skilled and a high degree of hygiene is vital. After colonic irrigation, careful dietary supplementation with vitamins, minerals, and probiotics, acidophilus, for example, is important.

a result of infection, food poisoning, or anxiety and stress. It is normally self-correcting but it can lead to a temporary loss of bowel control (fecal incontinence).

Warning: See a doctor if the diarrhea lasts more than 48 hours (24 hours in children), if there is blood or mucus in the stools, or the diarrhea is accompanied by vomiting.

Dietary and nutritional therapies
Drink plenty of water to avoid dehydration. To replace lost fluids and salts, dissolve 1 teaspoon of salt and 8 teaspoons of sugar in 3½ cups (1 liter) water and drink 1¾ cups (500 ml) every hour and eat no solid food until the diarrhea goes. Reintroduce bland foods gradually. Eating live yogurt, drinking the water that rice has been boiled in, and taking probiotic (acidophilus) capsules 3 times a day can all help.

Herbal medicine
Peppermint tea helps, as do agrimony, plantain, and geranium, or goldenseal.

Homeopathy
Arsenicum alb 6c, *Pulsatilla* 6c, and *Causticum* 6c may be beneficial. Individual prescription from a qualified therapist is advisable.

Massage and aromatherapy
A hot bath with 4–5 drops each of juniper, peppermint, and geranium oils can help. Or gently massage a blend of tea tree, peppermint, sandalwood, and geranium oils into the abdomen and lower back (5 drops each with a little carrier oil). ▶

The acupressure point known as Stomach 25 can help resolve diarrhea. Press in the abdomen very firmly at a point three fingers' width on either side of the navel.

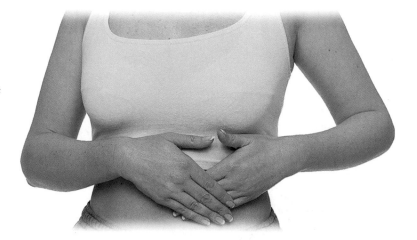

Digestive and urinary pain

GASTROENTERITIS

Severe inflammation of the stomach and intestines, usually as the result of a bacterial infection from contaminated food or water, is called gastroenteritis. It causes diarrhea, severe intestinal pain, fever, headache and fatigue. It often occurs when people are travelling abroad. Sensible precautions include drinking only bottled water, refusing drinks with ice cubes, washing and peeling fruit, and avoiding salads and foods that may have been kept warm for a long time.

Warning: The condition can be serious; avoid dehydration (see Naturopathy below). Conventional medical help should be sought if symptoms are severe and last for any length of time. An adult should see a doctor if the symptoms last more than 48 hours. Always see a doctor immediately if symptoms appear in children under 12 or the elderly. Severe cases may need antibiotics.

Naturopathy

A fast is recommended but keep taking liquids, especially water with added sea salt and sugar, or honey, if diarrhea is severe and prolonged (see p. 151). Follow the advice given for diarrhea.

IRRITABLE BOWEL SYNDROME

Irritable bowel syndrome or IBS ("syndrome" means it is a collection of symptoms of unknown cause) used to be called spastic colon and, though no longer used, the term explains the condition better. The colon muscles go into unpredictable spasm causing abdominal pain and cramps, bloating, back pain, flatulence, lethargy, headache,

---

APPENDICITIS

Appendicitis is inflammation of the appendix, a vestigial organ in a corner of the colon. Symptoms are pain which starts centrally but settles in the lower right abdomen, where the appendix is situated. The problem is potentially, though rarely, life-threatening if untreated, because it can lead to peritonitis – inflammation of the peritoneum, the membrane lining the walls of the abdomen. Always see a doctor immediately if appendicitis is suspected. In severe cases, an infected appendix may have to be removed by surgery.

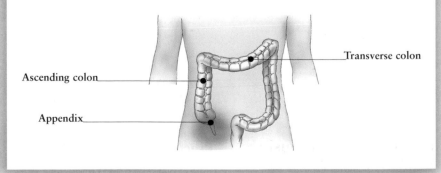

Ascending colon

Appendix

Transverse colon

fatigue, and diarrhea alternating with constipation. The problem is common and its incidence is increasing. No one is sure why, but diet and stress are widely believed to be to blame. The problem can come and go but once it starts it tends to be recurring and long lasting.

Dietary and nutritional therapies
A healthy, wholefood diet is essential, with regular exercise and stress control. Checking for food intolerances with an experienced therapist is also advised.

Relaxation therapies
Relaxation exercises, visualization, biofeedback and meditation are all helpful (see pp. 46–51).

Other therapies
Treatments useful for constipation and diarrhea (herbal medicine, massage and aromatherapy, acupressure and reflexology) can also help IBS (see pp. 150–151). An initial consultation with a qualified therapist is advisable.

DIVERTICULITIS
Diverticulitis is the inflammation of small pouches which appear in the wall of hollow organs, especially the intestines. It is one result of chronic constipation and irregular bowel movement.

Warning: An infected diverticulum may perforate and lead to peritonitis. Seek medical advice.

Dietary and nutritional therapies
Treat as for constipation (see pp. 150).

INFLAMMATORY BOWEL DISEASE
IBD is a blanket description for a range of disorders that occur in both the small and large intestines, including excessive flatulence (gas), ulcerative colitis and Crohn's disease (enteritis).

Colitis occurs in the large intestine, or colon, and its cause is uncertain, but not eating enough fiber and excessive stress may be partly to blame. It can cause diarrhea and pain and sometimes mucus and blood in the stools. Crohn's disease, in the small intestine, is the result of recurrent inflammation and is more serious since it can impede the absorption of nutrients from food, causing fever, diarrhea and weight loss, as well as pain.

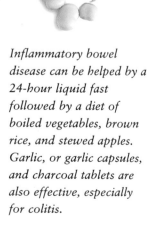

Dietary and nutritional therapies
Eat a healthy diet (see caption right) and avoid dairy products, sugar and refined and processed foods. Check for food intolerances through an experienced therapist.

Herbal medicine
Slippery elm taken twice a day and regular teas of lemon balm and chamomile are said to help.

Other therapies
Reflexology (as for constipation, p. 150) and homeopathy (as for diarrhea, p. 150), but consult a qualified therapist first. Relaxation therapies, as described for irritable bowel syndrome (above).

Practitioner therapies
- Cranial osteopathy
- Psychotherapy and counseling ▶

Find out more	
Digestive system	20
Nutritional therapy	33
Diarrhea	150

Inflammatory bowel disease can be helped by a 24-hour liquid fast followed by a diet of boiled vegetables, brown rice, and stewed apples. Garlic, or garlic capsules, and charcoal tablets are also effective, especially for colitis.

Digestive and urinary pain

Urinary tract infection

UTI, or urinary tract infection, is inflammation of part of the urinary tract, particularly the bladder, ureters, and kidneys. Urethritis (or nonspecific urethritis) is inflammation of the urethra. These infections result in pain on urinating, sometimes accompanied by blood or pus; severe headaches; and fever with shivering attacks.

Urinary tract infection is more common in women than in men and may result from bruising during sex. Urethritis is a bacterial infection, and is usually the result of a sexually transmitted disease. Nonspecific urethritis may be viral, or may result from sexual activity. In men, the condition is likely to be caused by bacterial infection from a sexual disease.

The condition needs medical attention but it can be treated as for cystitis below. Antibiotics may be necessary to treat urinary tract infection if the resulting pain is severe.

Warning: Untreated urinary tract infection can be dangerous. Seek medical attention as soon as possible.

Dietary and nutritional therapies

Drink plenty of water (6–8 glasses a day) and do not drink coffee, tea, alcohol, or acidic fruit juices. Barley water is effective (5 cups a day) and taking supplements of vitamin C (1 g a day) also helps.

Herbal medicine

Taking 2 drops of tea tree oil in a glass of warm water can be beneficial, as can regular teas of chamomile, yarrow, couch grass, buchu, and cornsilk.

Cranberry juice is a popular remedy for preventing cystitis, and increasing numbers of people attest to its effectiveness.

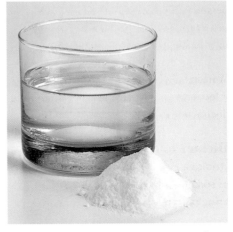

Drinking a solution of bicarbonate of soda is a simple and rapid way to relieve the pain that accompanies cystitis.

Cystitis

A form of urinary tract infection, cystitis is inflammation of the bladder caused by bacterial infection. It is relatively common —particularly among adult women (though both men and children can be affected also)—and tends to recur once it starts. Symptoms, which can range from mild to severe, include pain or a burning sensation on passing urine, a frequent need to urinate, feeling that the bladder is still full after urination, and occasionally, blood in the urine. The urine may also have a strong odor. In severe cases there can be accompanying fever and backache.

The causes of cystitis are many but include poor hygiene, inflammation caused as a reaction to chemicals in clothing and toiletries, and—commonly among women—sexual intercourse. It may also be due to a sexually transmitted disease, or caused by massaging the urethra during sex, which may introduce bacteria into the bladder. Other causes include incomplete emptying of the bladder, and stones or foreign bodies in the bladder. Pay particular attention to personal hygiene and abstain from penetrative sex. A number of remedies may hasten recovery and ease pain.

Warning: Cystitis may lead to kidney infection which can be serious. Consult a doctor if symptoms persist.

Dietary and nutritional therapies

Drinking half a teaspoon of bicarbonate of soda dissolved in warm water can bring pain relief in 20 minutes. Plain live

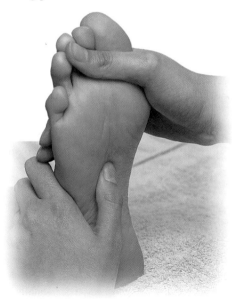

Reflexology treatment for cystitis includes massaging the areas on the foot that correspond to the kidneys and bladder.

yogurt applied generously to the genitals also helps. To prevent an attack, eat as healthy a diet as possible, especially one that is high in fresh vegetables and fruit, but avoid acidic fruits.

Cranberry juice is said to be an excellent preventive. Also drink plenty of fresh, preferably filtered water (6–8 glasses a day), and cut out coffee and all alcohol during an attack.

Naturopathy

Alternating warm and cold baths—the warm at body temperature—for half an hour can help. To help prevent attacks, always choose cotton underwear.

If you suffer from frequent bouts of cystitis try sitz bathing. This involves alternatively sitting in hot water up to your hips with your feet in cold water (and vice versa). It is not recommended for those with high blood pressure or a weak heart.

Herbal medicine

Chamomile tea is effective at the first sign of an attack and pain can be relieved by taking teas of cumin, coriander, and fennel (a cup 3 times a day). Regular teas of marigold, yarrow, cornsilk, and St. John's wort may help, as may couch grass and buchu. Echinacea, either as a liquid or as capsules, is good for any infection.

Homeopathy

Take *Cantharis* 6c and *Staphysagria* 6c hourly while symptoms last.

Acupressure/massage

Massaging and applying pressure to the lower abdomen at a point immediately over the bladder can soothe symptoms.

Aromatherapy

Three or four drops of essential oils of sandalwood, juniper, lavender, or bergamot mixed with a carrier oil and used as described above can ease pain and discomfort. Or add the oils to a bath.

Reflexology

Manipulate the center of the sole and in a diagonal line to each heel (the kidneys and bladder). Also try the center of the pad of the big toes (pituitary gland). ▶

Find out more

Dietary therapy	30
Aromatherapy	36
Herbal medicine	60

Digestive and urinary pain

HIATAL HERNIA

In a hiatal (or diaphragmatic) hernia part of the stomach slips back up through the opening in the diaphragm through which the gullet passes to reach the stomach. The usual cause is being overweight. Symptoms include pain—known as heartburn—behind the breastbone, difficulty in swallowing, bleeding, and regurgitation, particularly when lying down or stooping. This can cause choking if gastric juices from the stomach run back into the gullet. Corrective surgery used to be the normal treatment but this is now rarely performed.

Naturopathy

The problem can be self-correcting, especially if surplus weight is shed and a healthy diet eaten in moderate amounts. Sleeping with the head higher than the feet, or even sleeping in an armchair, can bring immediate relief. Treatments for ulcers (see below) may also be effective.

Yoga/Alexander technique

Many of the special breathing techniques and postures in yoga can help, as can the postural reeducation taught in the Alexander technique.

Practitioner therapies

- Osteopathy
- Chiropractic

ULCERS

Peptic ulcers occur in either the stomach or the duodenum. More specifically, ulcers in the stomach are gastric ulcers; those in the duodenum are duodenal ulcers. They are the most likely cause of severe recurring or chronic pain in the stomach and are usually preceded by inflammation (gastritis).

It is now known that about 90 percent of peptic ulcers are caused by the bacterium *Helicobacter pylori*. This means that most ulcers are cured by a

---

TWO TYPES OF HIATAL HERNIA

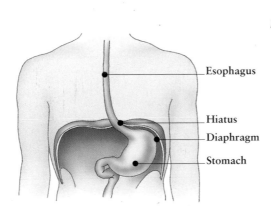

- Esophagus
- Hiatus
- Diaphragm
- Stomach

In a hiatal hernia a small loop of the stomach passes up through the hiatus, a small opening in the diaphragm. In a sliding hernia, the stomach enters the chest cavity; in a paraesophageal hernia, the stomach rests beside the esophagus.

Sliding hiatal hernia

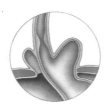

Paraesophageal hiatal hernia

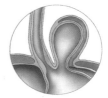

combination of antibiotics and a drug to reduce stomach acid production.

Peptic ulcers are more common in men than women. They are often aggravated by stress and anxiety combined with poor eating and drinking habits. This can cause a painful cavity in the walls of the protective mucus lining between the two organs. Gastric pain can cover an area on the stomach about the size of a hand and normally comes on after eating. Duodenal pain and tenderness is normally less acute, not so closely linked to eating and is only the size of a fingertip.

Warning: Ulcers may cause bleeding and perforation with peritonitis. Always seek medical advice.

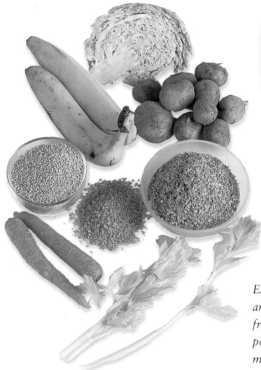

Eating whole-grain cereals and drinking juice made from cabbage, banana, potato, carrot, or celery may help relieve ulcers.

Dietary therapy

Radical changes in diet and lifestyle—including fasting—can successfully cure the problem, but a high degree of self-discipline is essential. Drinks such as tea, coffee, and alcohol, and all spicy food should be eliminated entirely, as should smoking. Instead eat brown rice, millet, buckwheat, rye, and whole-wheat together with whey concentrate and fresh-pressed juice drinks. Juices of raw potato, carrot, celery, cabbage, and bananas are recommended.

Stress management therapies

Because stress contributes to the formation of ulcers, it is essential to keep any sources of stress under control. Practice progressive muscular relaxation regularly, followed by visualization, biofeedback, and meditation. Appropriate yoga and t'ai chi exercises are also powerful antistressors if practiced regularly. General exercise will be beneficial, too.

Herbal medicine

A teaspoon of oil of St. John's wort (hypericum) taken morning and night is effective against gastritis, while a tablespoon of aloe vera juice extract taken in a glass of warm water three times a day helps ulcers. Licorice and bilberry juice, at full strength, is also said to be effective. Alternatively, drink marsh mallow, coriander, or lemon balm teas.

Homeopathy

Remedies likely to help include *Arsenicum alb, Argentum nit, Lycopodium,* and *Nux vomica* but individual prescription from an experienced homeopath is advisable.

Practitioner therapies

• Acupuncture for pain relief
• Chinese herbal medicine for pain relief
• Hypnotherapy to help deal with stress and to learn to relax

Digestive and urinary pain

KIDNEY STONES

These are hard deposits of chemical salts that lodge in the kidneys (and sometimes the ureter). Causes include a deficiency of vitamin A, reduced citrate (citric acid salt) in the urine, kidney infection, a blockage in the urinary system, or a metabolic dysfunction. Prolonged inactivity may increase the amount of calcium in the urine, also leading to stone formation.

Symptoms are constant if mild pain in the lower back on one side. Ultrasound disintegrates the stones and allows them to flush away naturally, without surgery.

Warning: Severe pain may mean a stone has passed from the kidney into the ureter. Seek immediate medical intervention.

Naturopathy

A compress of Epsom salts applied over the kidneys and abdomen for 10–15 minutes as often as needed can relieve pain. Or try a hot bath with Epsom salts.

Kidney stones form when crystals of calcium and other chemicals in the urine make hard deposits in the kidney. When a stone passes into the ureter it can cause extreme pain and difficulty in passing urine.

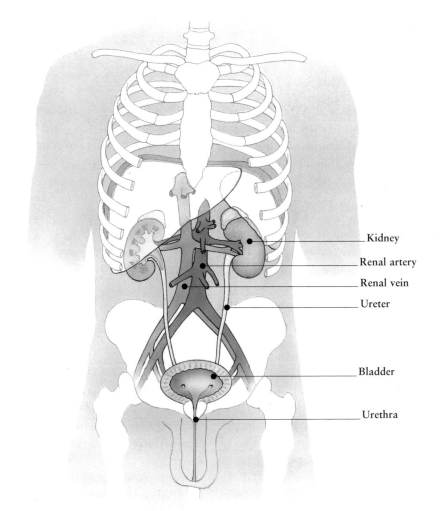

Kidney

Renal artery

Renal vein

Ureter

Bladder

Urethra

Dietary therapy

Drink lots of fresh water and cut down on dairy products and other calcium-rich foods, such as chocolate, strawberries, rhubarb, grapes, spinach, and beet. A daily dose of a little cider vinegar or lemon juice in warm water with honey is said to be effective in dissolving stones.

Herbal medicine

Regular tinctures of gravel root, stone root, parsley, and wild carrot are said to help dissolve stones over a period of time. An alternative is to drink nettle tea regularly (3 times a day).

Homeopathy

Berberis 6c, *Sarsaparilla* 6c, *Magnesia phos* 6c, and *Calcarea* 6c are said to help relieve pain from a blocked ureter but see a qualified therapist first.

Practitioner therapies

• Acupuncture for pain relief
• Chinese herbal medicine

GALLSTONES

Formed of cholesterol and calcium salts, gallstones are mineral deposits in the gallbladder. They may cause digestive problems and infection of the gallbladder, which may lead to perforation and even peritonitis.

They are painful and surgery may be necessary if the stones block the flow of bile from the liver. Apart from pain, felt in the upper abdomen and right shoulder (referred pain), symptoms that stones have passed into the bile duct include jaundice, heartburn, and fever.

See a doctor if symptoms are severe. Ultrasound disintegrates the stones harmlessly and allows them to flush away naturally without surgery.

Dietary and nutritional therapies

A liver flush is the favored treatment to remove gallstones. For 6 days eat and drink nothing but whole foods and apples with plenty of raw apple juice. On the morning of the seventh day drink a cup of a mixture of olive oil and lemon juice (half a cup of each). This is claimed to flush the stones out by stimulating a flood of bile from the liver.

Foods that are good for the liver, and therefore the gallbladder, include globe artichokes, chicory, radishes, endives, and dandelion leaves (excellent in salad). Drink noncarbonated water, cut out all animals fats and dairy products, and supplement with vitamin C.

Herbal medicine

Drinking 2–3 cups of centaury tea every day for 4 weeks may clear stones. Or mix two parts marsh mallow with one part each of balmony, boldo, fringetree bark, and goldenseal and drink it as a tea three times a day. Stone root, gentian, rosemary, and dandelion may also help, but you should consult a qualified herbalist for an individual prescription. Herbs for gallstones are not recommended during pregnancy.

Aromatherapy

Vaporizing Scotch pine essential oil in a burner can help to relieve pain.

Reflexology

Pressing a point in the center of the arch on the sole of the left foot (corresponding to the gallbladder) for 10–15 seconds each day may help.

Practitioner therapies

• Acupuncture for pain relief
• Chinese herbal medicine for pain relief

Find out more

Herbal medicine	60
Acupuncture	68
Reflexology	74

Reproductive system pain: general

Because women have a monthly cycle, they may experience pain in their reproductive system more frequently than men; men have problems of their own, often later in life. Both sexes, however, are affected by sexually transmitted diseases (STDs).

The microorganism Chlamydia trachomatis, *which causes chlamydia, has characteristics of both a virus and a bacterium. Chlamydia may be spread through vaginal or anal sex, and is usually treated with antibiotics.*

Pubic lice (crabs), genital herpes, nonspecific urethritis (NSU), may prove relatively harmless. Other STDs, however, are serious. Accurate diagnosis by a medical practitioner is vital if you suspect an STD. AIDS sufferers may benefit from therapies that boost the immune system and ease symptoms. Counseling is also essential.

Warning: Gonorrhea, syphilis, and AIDS are suitable for treatment only under proper medical supervision.

GENITAL HERPES

A viral infection caused by *Herpes simplex* (also responsible for cold sores), genital herpes is characterized by painful sores on the penis or in the vagina. These form blisters, burst, and dry.

Naturopathy/herbal medicine

Wash the affected parts with salt water (1 tsp of salt to 1 pint of water). Alternatively, apply tea tree oil to the sores or blisters and witch hazel to dry them.

CHLAMYDIA

Chlamydia is an infection caused by the parasite *Chlamydia trachomatis,* which lodges in the urethra and, in women, the vagina. Symptoms include a sore vagina, pain during sex, a tender cervix, the urge to urinate, and an irritating discharge.

Warning: If left untreated chlamydia can spread to other parts of the reproductive system, causing pelvic inflammatory disease (PID), infertility, and long-term debility. Medical treatment is essential.

Naturopathy

Colonic irrigation by an experienced practitioner, followed by supplementation with *Lactobacillus,* is recommended.

Dietary and nutritional therapy

Eat a healthy diet (more fresh fruit and vegetables, less sugar, processed food, and alcohol) and take supplements of vitamins A, C, and E, and zinc.

Herbal medicine

A daily vaginal douche of calendula, goldenseal, and echinacea is effective. Insert plain yogurt on a tampon in the evening.

Practitioner therapies
• Homeopathy

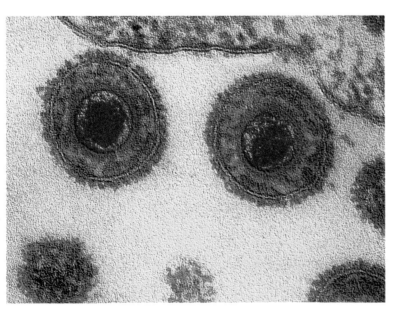

HERNIA FIRST AID

Attempt to return the hernia to where it came from by gentle but firm inward pressure, then use a support or truss to hold the tissues in place. Do not truss a hernia you cannot return manually and that has become trapped. To help prevent a recurrence, take care not to strain.

A trapped or "strangulated" hernia can be dangerous and requires surgery to correct. Surgery is almost always necessary if the problem recurs frequently.

Hernia

Usually taken to mean a rupture in the groin in men, a hernia may occur in any part of the abdomen where the contents, mainly the intestines, push through a weakness in the abdominal wall and cause inflammation and swelling.

Men are more prone than women to hernia in the groin. The condition is often painful and debilitating, especially if the protrusion pushes into the scrotum. Straining to lift heavy weights or to make bowel movements are the most common causes of hernia.

Warning: Although a hernia is reducible, it will always slip out again if not trussed. Always seek medical advice.

Find out more

Psychotherapy	76
Urinary tract infection	154
Hiatal hernia	156

Lifting heavy weights
When you lift using your back you put yourself at risk of back problems and of hernia. Always bend the knees when lifting and tighten your abdominal muscles.

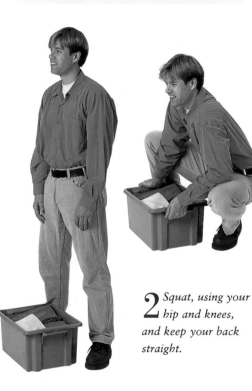

1 *Stand close to the object with your feet on either side of it.*

2 *Squat, using your hip and knees, and keep your back straight.*

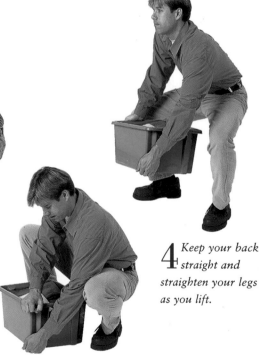

3 *Lift an edge slightly so that you can get one hand underneath.*

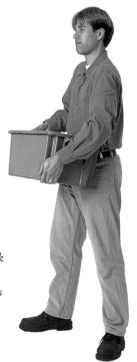

4 *Keep your back straight and straighten your legs as you lift.*

5 *Keep the weight close to your body when carrying it.*

Reproductive system pain: men

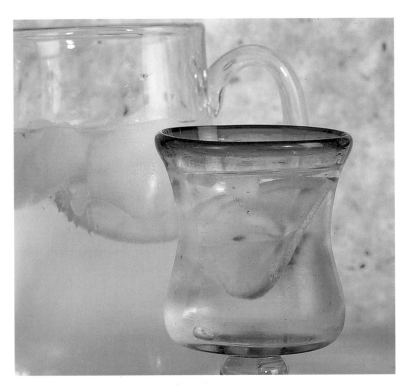

For prostatitis, drink plenty of water. This avoids dehydration, which places stress on the prostate, and encourages frequent urination, relieving congestion.

PROSTATE PROBLEMS

Prostatitis is inflammation of the prostate gland due to an infection. The walnut-sized prostate gland lies immediately below the bladder and is involved in the manufacture of semen.

Prostatism is the natural enlargement of the gland with age (especially over 50), which restricts the working of the bladder.

Symptoms of prostatitis are similar to those of the flu, with pain, particularly in the lower back, shivering, and fever.

Warning: Untreated prostatitis can lead to inflammation of other parts of the genito-urinary system, including the testes. Medical advice is essential.

Naturopathy

Drink plenty of fluids, preferably water (but not tea, coffee, or alcohol), and urinate frequently, making sure the

bladder is as empty as possible. Sit in a waist-deep hot bath for about 10 minutes, with your knees bent and a cold face cloth on your forehead.

Afterward, rub down your lower half with a cold towel and hold it between your legs for a few seconds to cool the area. Some therapists recommend regular ejaculation and massage of the prostate to relieve pressure from enlargement. Seek advice from your doctor if you wish to self massage.

Regular exercise, particularly walking and cycling, also helps.

Dietary and nutritional therapies

Avoid spicy and fatty foods and take daily supplements of vitamins C, E, and B-complex, as well as zinc and magnesium. Regular supplementation with fish oils, olive oil, and evening primrose oil can also help. Try juices of carrot, celery, watercress, and horseradish; carrot, beet, cucumber, radish, and garlic; and pumpkin.

Herbal medicine

Teas of dandelion, saw palmetto, fygeum, horsetail, and couch grass are said to be effective. Tinctures of pipsissewa, echinacea, *Staphysagria,* and *Pulsatilla* may also be beneficial, but individual prescription from a qualified herbal therapist is advisable.

Massage and aromatherapy

Massaging with or inhaling the essential oils of lavender, cypress, and thyme may be beneficial.

Reflexology

Massage a point midway between the ankle bone and the heel on the inside of the foot. The same point also benefits the uterus in women.

Practitioner therapies

- Acupuncture and Chinese herbal medicine
- Colonic irrigation

IMPOTENCE

The inability to achieve or maintain an erection, impotence can be physical—as a result of illness or infection—but is often psychological. A physical problem can usually be detected fairly easily by a family doctor, especially if illness is involved (some medicines and drugs can cause impotence, for example). But if there is no obvious physical reason, the cause is most likely psychological. A combination of treatments that simultaneously promote both relaxation and desire is most effective.

Partner therapy

Recruiting your sexual partner is important. Agree to caresses and cuddles without any other expectations. Do not have intercourse until you feel relaxed and confident about it. Also make sure the circumstances for lovemaking are relaxed and unhurried.

Naturopathy

A daily cold bath or a sitz bath, where you sit alternately in hot and cold water, can be effective if done regularly. Frequent exercise is beneficial.

Massage and aromatherapy

Being massaged all over the body (except the genitals) with the essential oils of ylang ylang, jasmine, rose, sandalwood, jojoba, or patchouli—all renowned aphrodisiacs—is both mentally relaxing and physically stimulating. Massaging the neck and head, including the scalp, with rosemary can also help.

Dietary and nutritional therapies

Aside from eating and drinking healthily (plenty of fresh fruit and vegetables and not too much alcohol), foods rich in vitamin C and zinc are beneficial. Taking a regular supplement that contains vitamin C and zinc can also help.

Herbal medicine

Teas of saw palmetto and fygeum are said to be beneficial.

Relaxation therapies

Muscle relaxation exercises, visualization, meditation, and biofeedback can all help overcome the effects of psychological strain that may lie behind impotence and reassert a more positive frame of mind.

Practitioner therapies

- Psychotherapy and counseling (including sex therapy)
- Hypnotherapy

Find out more	
Dietary therapy	30
Meditation	48
Psychotherapy	76

Vitamin C and zinc are helpful in cases of impotence. Broccoli, red peppers, and blackcurrants are good sources of vitamin C, while shellfish, sardines, pumpkin seeds, chicken, and brown rice are rich in zinc.

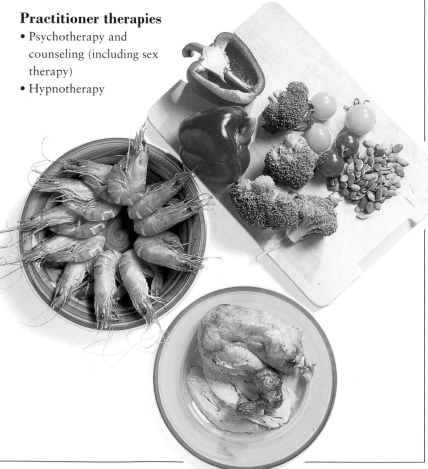

Reproductive system pain: women

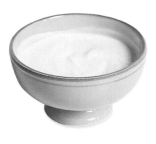

Applying natural live yogurt to the vagina provides effective relief for the discomfort caused by a yeast infection.

VAGINITIS

An infection usually caused by *Candida albicans* (thrush), vaginitis results in inflammation of the vagina. Other causes include infection by the parasite *Trichomonas vaginalis*, and transmission during sex, if a man is a symptomless carrier. It is more common after menopause when the lining of the vagina thins as a result of reduced estrogen production, which makes bruising and infection more likely. Symptoms are soreness and itching and sometimes a discharge with blood. Antibiotics may be necessary to clear the infection.

The form known as nonspecific vaginitis occurs when normal vaginal bacteria multiply for no apparent reason, causing a fishy-smelling vaginal discharge.

Herbal medicine

Regular herbal douches with hypericum (St. John's wort) and calendula are an effective treatment: mix 10 drops of each of the mother tinctures in about 17 fl oz (500 ml) of boiled warm water.

An alternative is a bath with several drops of lavender essential oil in it (avoid chemical soaps and detergents). Aloe vera tincture (diluted) or gel is also effective.

If the cause is being too dry for sex—a problem for many postmenopausal women—ensure your partner uses a water-based lubricating gel. If inflammation is present, try a drop or two of tea tree oil in a neutral carrier oil.

VAGINAL YEAST INFECTION (CANDIDA)

The vaginal infection known as candida or candidiasis is caused by an overgrowth of the yeastlike fungus *Candida albicans*. This is characterized by severe itching in the vagina and vulva, a thick white discharge from the vagina, fatigue, headache, and aching limbs. It can make having sex and urinating painful.

Candida albicans is a normal part of human flora—the minute organisms that live in the body, particularly the mouth, vagina, and intestines. Normally its growth is checked by bacteria in these

---

VAGINISMUS

In vaginismus, the vaginal muscles go into spasm, blocking the entrance to the vagina and making penetrative sex painful or impossible.

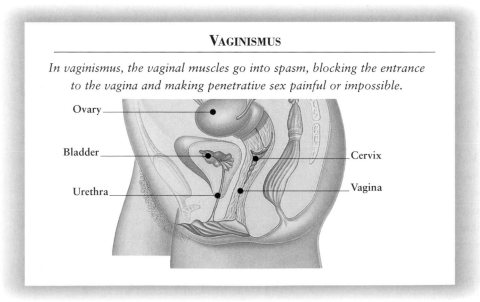

areas. If these are compromised—by a course of antibiotics, for example—*Candida albicans* will multiply.

Warning: Vaginal yeast infections require specialist help, usually treatment with antifungal drugs. Consult your doctor.

Naturopathy/nutritional therapy

To ease itching, place natural live yogurt into the vagina—cover a tampon and insert it—and leave it there for at least an hour.

Eat 2–3 bowls a day of natural live yogurt supplemented with two *Lactobacillus acidophilus* capsules. Avoid sugar, other refined carbohydrates, and alcohol (yeasts feed on them) and eat plenty of salads with garlic, fresh fruit, and whole grains. Avoid intercourse during an attack.

Aromatherapy

Douche with 2–3 drops of oils of tea tree, bergamot, and myrrh; or lavender, bergamot, and rose in 3½ cups (1 liter) of warm water. Tea tree oil can be applied directly as an antifungal and antiseptic.

Herbal medicine

A warm compress of goldenseal, myrrh, or chamomile can relieve symptoms.

Practitioner therapies

• Homeopathy

VAGINISMUS

Vaginismus is a painful spasm of the vagina, in which the vagina involuntarily tightens. If it occurs during sex, it makes intercourse difficult, if not impossible, without pain. Vaginismus may be psychological, but chronic vaginitis can cause painful intercourse, which may lead to the condition.

Vaginismus is often associated with low sexual response but it is not the same: a woman may want penetrative sex but be unable to relax her vagina for reasons she is often unaware of and cannot control.

Partner therapy

The help of a sympathetic sexual partner and setting the scene for relaxing, trusting, and unhurried sex are often successful.

Try a hot, waist-deep bath by candlelight, with a glass of wine if you like, followed by masturbation to orgasm. Teaching your partner how to do it for you can also be effective, as can a massage.

Practitioner therapies

• Counseling or psychotherapy
• Hypnotherapy

Find out more

Massage	56
Hypnotherapy	77
Chlamydia	160

A massage from a caring partner with neroli, ylang ylang, or rose oil is a sensual experience and can help create an atmosphere of love and trust. This, in turn, may help prevent vaginismus.

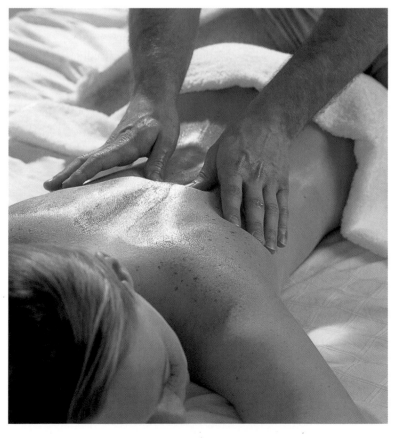

Reproductive system pain: women

PREMENSTRUAL SYNDROME

Premenstrual syndrome (PMS) describes a collection of symptoms that result from changes in hormone levels just before menstruation. PMS causes a range of symptoms, including depression, tension headaches, irritability, mood swings, food cravings, feelings of being bloated, and tenderness in the breasts.

Reactions to PMS vary from mild to extremely severe and they differ between individuals as well as from month to month for any one person.

Naturopathy

Regular outdoor exercise and a warm bath with lemongrass essential oil is relaxing and calming.

Dietary and nutritional therapies

Eat a healthy diet with plenty of salads and leafy green vegetables and cut down on dairy products, sugar, salt, caffeine, and alcohol.

Supplementing with vitamins C, B-complex, and E, as well as the minerals zinc, magnesium, and iron, and a balance of essential fatty acids (2 EPA to 1 GLA) can help (see p.143).

Herbal medicine

A tea blend containing chaste tree berries (*Agnus castus*), Mexican yam, ginseng, licorice, fennel, kelp, black cohosh, and false unicorn may help. Drunk 3 times daily during the second half of the menstrual cycle for at least 3 months, the tea is said to regulate hormone levels.

A wide range of herbs is available for PMS symptoms such as depression and anxiety (borage, lemon balm); breast pain and tenderness (evening primrose); water retention (dandelion, cleavers); headaches (meadowsweet, willow bark); and

insomnia (chamomile). It is advisable, however, to see a qualified herbalist for individual prescription.

Reflexology

Apply pressure to the points on the soles of both feet said to be associated with PMS symptoms. Consult a qualified reflexologist who will be able to relieve your particular symptoms.

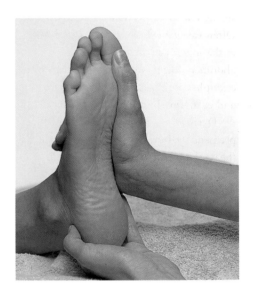

In reflexology, the big toe, instep, and center of the foot are said to be associated with premenstrual syndrome.

Relaxation therapy

Learning to handle stress and relax using relaxation techniques is an important part of PMS treatment.

Practitioner therapies

- Acupuncture and Traditional Chinese Medicine
- Homeopathy
- Counseling and psychotherapy
- Hypnotherapy
- Creative arts therapy

MENSTRUAL PAIN

Known technically as dysmenorrhea, menstrual pain usually means cramps experienced in the lower abdomen during menstruation. The pain is the result of excessive contractions to expel the lining of the womb at menstruation. This is usually due to an overproduction of the hormonelike substances called prostaglandins that promote the contractions. Too many result in such strong contractions that they cause pain. Often this is no more than a dull ache in the lower part of the back or abdomen, but in severe cases, it can be a cramplike pain accompanied by nausea and even diarrhea.

Dysmenorrhea is different from premenstrual syndrome and menorrhagia (heavy bleeding). The latter is usually caused by normally nonpainful and harmless fibroids (growths) in the uterus. Painful periods can sometimes also be caused by inflammation of the uterus (see box on uterine pain, p. 168).

Naturopathy
Exercise and having a hot bath with caraway seed oil in it are beneficial.

Dietary and nutritional therapies
Healthy eating and drinking will help, particularly reducing intake of animal fats, saturated oils, and salt, and eating plenty of fresh fruit, vegetables, whole grains, seeds, nuts, and legumes.

A good multivitamin and mineral tablet containing vitamin B_6 and magnesium will also help, as will evening primrose oil with vitamin E.

Herbal medicine
The Chinese herb *dong quai* (*Angelica sinensis*) provides effective relief from menstrual pain. Raspberry leaf tea and ginger are also said to help.

Acupressure
Points on the abdomen, lower back, and legs are useful for pain relief. See a qualified practitioner.

Yoga
The cobra posture is particularly helpful for menstrual pain; other useful postures are the cat and the bow.

Relaxation therapy
Learning to relax is beneficial for all forms of menstrual pain, and biofeedback has been shown to be effective. ▶

Find out more	
Yoga	40
Relaxation	46
Essential fatty acids	143

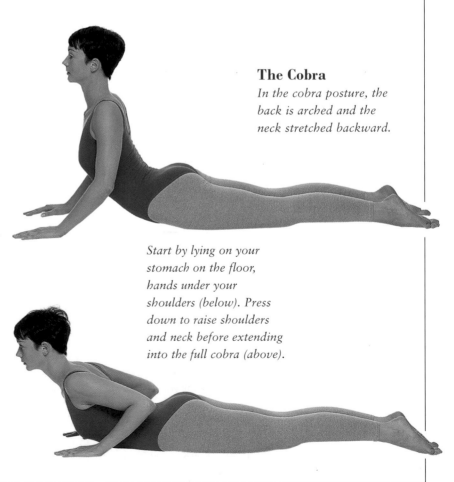

The Cobra
In the cobra posture, the back is arched and the neck stretched backward.

Start by lying on your stomach on the floor, hands under your shoulders (below). Press down to raise shoulders and neck before extending into the full cobra (above).

Reproductive system pain: women

PROLAPSE

Prolapse of the womb or uterus usually results from a combination of age and being overweight, often as a result of earlier pregnancy. Slack muscles allow the pelvic organs to sag, causing aching sensations and feelings of heaviness in the lower back and abdomen, as well as incontinence and constipation.

Warning: Severe prolapse may lead to urinary obstruction and infection. Seek medical advice.

Naturopathy

Getting exercise and losing weight are essential. Exercises to tone up the muscles of the pelvis are the knee hug and the pelvic lift which must be carried out regularly over a period of time for real improvement. If symptoms do not improve, surgery may have to be considered.

Dietary therapy

A high-fiber diet relieves constipation, a common symptom of womb prolapse.

Symptoms of a prolapsed womb often include constipation. Eat foods that are high in fiber, including whole-wheat bread, cereals with bran, and fresh fruit, and be sure to drink plenty of water.

Herbal medicine

The herbs black cohosh, raspberry leaf, and chaste tree are reputed to tone the uterus. They should be drunk either as tinctures diluted in water or as teas. A mixture of these herbs combined with wild yam can relieve cramps.

PELVIC INFLAMMATORY DISEASE

When one or more organs of the female reproductive system become infected or inflamed, pelvic inflammatory disease (PID) results. The organs affected can include the ovaries, Fallopian tubes, uterus, and cervix. Symptoms of PID include severe abdominal pain, backache, fever, vaginal discharge, heavy or painful periods, pain or bleeding during sex, fatigue, and long-term debility.

Pelvic inflammatory disease can be caused by injury through sex, the intrauterine contraceptive device (IUD), endometriosis (see box below), sexually transmitted diseases, or abortion.

Warning: Antibiotics are likely to be necessary. PID can be extremely serious and medical assistance should be sought as a matter of urgency.

UTERINE PAIN

Uterine pain is normally the result of two conditions with similar sounding names, although they are different.

Endometritis is a rare but painful condition caused by inflammation of the walls of the uterus (endometrium), usually from bacterial infection after childbirth. Symptoms are pain in the lower part of the back and abdomen and erratic menstruation. Conventional treatment involves antibiotics and, if the problem recurs, dilatation and curettage (D&C) surgery. In endometriosis, uterine tissue grows outside the uterus and swells in normal response to the monthly hormone cycle, sometimes causing sudden pain. Both require medical treatment, but symptoms can be eased by the treatments for menstrual pain.

Naturopathy

Resting, eating a healthy diet, and taking hot baths, especially with the essential oils of cypress and lavender added, are recommended to alleviate symptoms.

Nutritional therapies

A good multivitamin and mineral supplement with vitamins A, B-complex, C, and E, zinc, magnesium, and selenium can help. Take the EPA and GLA essential fatty acids and, after antibiotics, *Lactobacillus acidophilus* (two capsules daily) to build up natural bacteria.

Acupressure

For abdominal cramps, apply pressure to a point just above the pubic bone, four fingers' width below the navel; and to a point on the edge of the shinbone, four fingers' widths above the inside ankle bone. **Do not use this point during pregnancy.**

Practitioner therapies

• Acupuncture
• Traditional Chinese medicine
• Homeopathy
• Herbal medicine

Find out more	
Dietary therapy	30
Herbal medicine	60
Menstrual pain	167

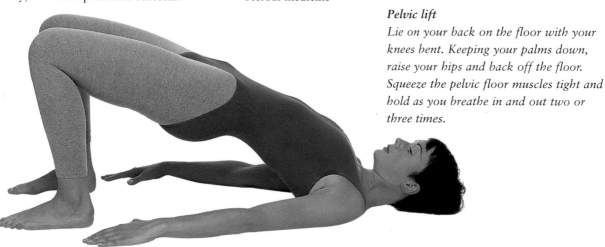

Pelvic lift
Lie on your back on the floor with your knees bent. Keeping your palms down, raise your hips and back off the floor. Squeeze the pelvic floor muscles tight and hold as you breathe in and out two or three times.

Knee hug
Lie on your back on the floor, then bring your knees up toward your chest. Grasp your knees with your hands and pull them toward you, pressing your knees against this force. Breathing in and out, clench the pelvic floor muscles, and hold the clench for two or three breaths.

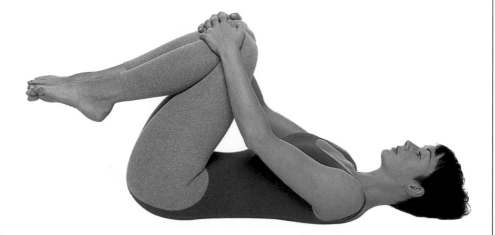

Pain due to cancer

*W*hen *rogue cells in the body start multiplying rapidly and abnormally, cancer is the result. The cancerous cells grow to such an extent that they interfere with the proper workings of the body. The reasons why this happens are not yet fully understood, but among likely culprits identified so far are poor eating habits, viral infection, stress, and environmental pollution.*

Cancer is a disease that is feared as much for its mysterious origins and unpredictable nature—which make it hard to treat successfully—as for its reputation for causing pain. In fact, most cancers do not cause pain—at least in the early stages. Some estimates have suggested that as few as half and no more than three-quarters of all those with cancer feel pain. Some cancers—liver cancer, for example—cause minimal pain even in the advanced stages. When pain is felt it is more usually the result of the cancerous growth pressing on a nerve or interfering with some other bodily function than from the cancer itself.

Effective treatment for pain requires combining various psychological and physical approaches to make maximum use of the body's potential to promote health using the mind and emotions. Self-help is possible in cancer to a greater extent than is commonly realized, especially with the positive assistance and support of family or friends.

Warning: The approaches described here complement conventional medical treatment for cancer pain; they are not alternatives to it. Up to 90 percent of cancer patients respond well to drug control of their pain; it is also known that cancer cells tend to grow less quickly when pain is well controlled. It is illegal in many countries for anyone who is not a medical doctor to treat cancer.

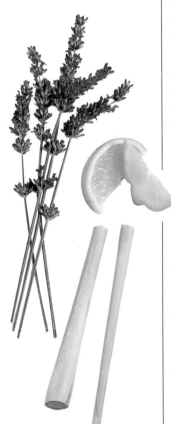

The refreshing scents of aromatherapy oils based on lemon, lemongrass, and lavender are said to soothe pain.

Electronic devices

TENS and other electronic pain-relieving devices counter cancer pain in exactly the same way as any other pain—by blocking the passage of pain messages to the brain and stimulating the release of endorphins. TENS devices can be prescribed by a doctor, but they are also widely available over the counter from specialist stores in most countries. Some manufacturers loan machines on a sale or return basis, so it is worth trying one out before you buy it.

Nutritional therapy

Vitamins and minerals do not have the painkilling properties of some herbs, but some are known to have distinct cancer-fighting qualities. They include the antioxidant vitamins A (preferably in the form of betacarotene), C, and E, and the minerals selenium, zinc, and manganese.

Massage with aromatherapy

Massaging with essential oils may be very helpful in controlling pain due to cancer, especially if you can find someone to do it for you. Essentials oils of geranium, jasmine, juniper, or Roman chamomile are commonly recommended.

It is advisable not to massage over the actual site of the tumor or where treatment has made the body tender or sore. Vaporizing essential oils of lemon, lemongrass, and/or lavender in a burner in the room may also help.

Reflexology

The same principle applies in the use of reflexology as with massage except that reflexology has the advantage that areas or organs of the body affected by tumors can be massaged indirectly via the feet. The same oils useful in massage can be used on the feet and, again, it is better if someone does the manipulating for you, making sure they use firm but not sharp pressure (thumbs are best for this) for 5–10 seconds at a time.

Acupressure

Acupressure, including shiatsu, follow on from the above two therapies in cancer pain relief. Applying finger, thumb, knuckle, or even whole hand pressure to points that relate to the area of the body affected can be very effective (see Acupressure, p. 38). Pressure should be steady and deep (though not painful) and last for about 20 seconds at a time.

Herbal medicine

A range of herbs can help in cancer pain depending on both the symptoms and the individual. Most important are red clover, Jamaican dogwood, bloodroot, Pacific Island potato, lady's slipper, skullcap, passionflower, and valerian. For nausea, ginger is helpful. But the advice of a qualified medical herbalist is essential to get the best treatment for your situation.

Homeopathy

Nux vomica (3c or 6c, taken three times daily for a month) is said to relieve discomfort, particularly nausea, caused by conventional cancer treatments such as chemotherapy.

Exercise

Swimming and walking can help reduce anxiety at the same time as building up the body's defenses.

Practitioner therapies

- Acupuncture
- Healing

Find out more	
Nutritional therapy	33
Aromatherapy	36
TENS	83

SUPPLEMENTS FOR CANCER

A complex supplement of 17 minerals developed in the early 1970s by a Hungarian doctor, Joseph Béres, claims to have dramatic pain-relieving effects in a wide range of conditions, including cancer. Called Béres Drops Plus, the combination claims to work by restoring the body's natural mineral balance. It is not widely available. Another controversial but more widely available supplement for cancer is ground shark cartilage. This claims to work over a period of some weeks by inhibiting and reducing the growth of cancer cells.

PSYCHOLOGICAL HELP

Psychological techniques provide ways of helping to deal with and overcome pain by harnessing the ability of the mind to influence the body. To alleviate cancer pain, it is important to concentrate on destressing the body, while promoting relaxation and positive thinking. Self-help techniques most helpful in overcoming pain in cancer are:
- *Meditation*
- *Autogenic training*
- *Visualization*
- *Creative arts therapy, especially music and painting*

Practitioner therapies that can help cultivate a positive mental attitude to help combat pain include:
- *Psychotherapy*
- *Counseling*
- *Assertiveness training*
- *Hypnotherapy*

Glossary

Acupuncture point - specific points along the meridians at which the flow of chi or qi, the fundamental life energy of the universe, can be stimulated.

Acute pain - a sudden pain, often the result of injury or infection.

Analgesic - pain-relieving substance or drug.

Asanas - specific yoga postures that gently stretch the body.

Atopic- inherited (used to describe allergies).

Chi (pronounced chee) - the fundamental life-energy of the universe, also known as qi and as prana in traditional Indian medicine.

Chronic - of long-term duration.

Endorphins - naturally occurring hormones that block the sensations of pain.

Endoscope - a device used in keyhole surgery to carry miniature tools and a camera to the precise area to be operated on.

Energy therapies - treatments that promote healing by manipulating the body's "energy force" to correct an imbalance. Homeopathy, reflexology, and shiatsu all follow this approach.

Epidural - an injection of painkilling drugs into the spinal canal in the lower back.

Essential oil - an aromatic liquid extracted from a plant, which aromatherapists believe contains the "life-force" of the plant.

Holistic therapy - an approach that considers the individual as a whole and encourages patients to take an active role in their treatment.

Meridian - one of 14 channels that run through the body carrying the life force, an energy known as qi or chi (pronounced chee).

Physical therapies - therapies that see pain as a symptom of a physical cause, which can be treated through the body, whether by nutrition, massage, acupuncture, or physiotherapy.

Prana - the fundamental life-energy of the universe in traditional Indian medicine. Also known as chi or qi in traditional Chinese medicine.

Psychological therapies - treatments that promote a positive attitude and encourage mental and physical relaxation. Examples include meditation, counseling, and hypnotherapy.

Referred pain - pain that originates in one part of the body but is actually felt in a different location.

Succussion - the process by which a homeopathic remedy is made more powerful or "potentized." Each time the remedy is diluted, it is shaken to imprint the energy of the original substance on molecules in the liquid. This shaking is known as succussion.

Tincture - an herbal remedy prepared by chopping or grinding a plant and soaking it in a solution of alcohol. The mixture is left to stand for several weeks, then the liquid is strained off and taken by mouth.

Tisane - an herbal remedy prepared in a similar manner to brewing tea. The herbs are infused in hot water in a teapot for about 10 minutes, then the liquid is poured off and drunk hot or cold.

Tsubo - special pressure point along a meridian, used in shiatsu.

Helpful organizations

ORGANIZATIONS IN THE U.S.A.

American Chronic Pain Association
P.O. Box 850
Rocklin, CA 95677
916-632-0922
www.theacpa.org

National Chronic Pain Outreach
Association
7979 Old Georgetown Road,
Suite 100
Bethesda, MD 20814
301-652-4948

American Association of
Acupuncture and Oriental Medicine
433 Front St.
Catasauqua, PA 18032
610-266-1433
www.aaom.org

American Academy of Medical
Acupuncture
5820 Wilshire Blvd, Suite 500
Los Angeles, CA 90036
323-937-5514
www.medicalacupuncture.org

North American Society of Teachers
of the Alexander Technique
P.O. Box 3992
Champagne, Il 61826
www.Alexandertech.com

Association for Applied
Psychophysiology and Biofeedback
10200 West 44th Avenue, suite 304
Wheat Ridge, CO 80033
303-422-8436
www.AAPB.org

National Center for Homeopathy
801 N. Fairfax Street, Suite 306
Alexandria, VA 22314
703-548-7792
www.healthy.net/nch/index.html

American Chiropractic Association
1701 Clarendon Boulevard
Arlington, VA 22209
703-276-8800
www.AMERCHIRO.org

American Botanical Council
P.O. Box 144345
Austin,TX 78714
512-331-8868
www.herbalgram.org

American Society of Clinical
Hypnosis
2200 East Devon Avenue, Suite 291
Des Plaines, IL 60018
312-645-9810

American Yoga Association
513 South Orange Avenue
Sarasota, FL 34236
941-953-5859
www.hindusamajtemple.org/ht/yoga
_assns.html

Feldenkrais Guild
P.O. Box 489
Albany, OR 97321
800-775-2118
www.feldenkrais.com

ORGANIZATIONS IN CANADA

Acupuncture Foundation of Canada
2131 Lawrence Avenue E, Suite 204
Scarborough, ON M1R 5G4
Tel: (416) 752-3988

Canadian Chiropractic Association
1396 Eglinton Avenue W
Toronto, ON M6C 2E4
Tel: (416) 781-5656

Reflexology Association of Canada
Box 110, 451 Turnberry Street
Brussels, ON N0G 1M0
Tel: (519) 887-9991

Canadian Association of
Homeopathic Physicians
10240A 152nd Street
Surrey, BC V3R 6N7
Tel: (604) 951-9987

Canadian Osteopathic Association
575 Waterloo Street
London, ON N6B 2R2
Tel: (519) 439-5521

The Canadian Association of Herbal
Practitioners
#400 - 1228 Kensington Road NW
Calgary, AB T2N 4P9
Tel: (403) 270-0936

Index

Acknowledgments

The publishers wish to acknowledge the invaluable contribution made to this book by Andrew Sydenham who took all the photographs except:

2 Tony Latham; 6 Camera Press; 9 Henry Arden; 10 Tony Stone; 13 The Stock Market; 17 Science Photo Library; 19 Science Photo Library; 27 Science Photo Library; 29 (top) The Stock Market; 34 Science Photo Library; 36 Camera Press; 38 Laura Wickenden; 39, Laura Wickenden; 40 Henry Arden; 41 Henry Arden; 43–45 Laura Wickenden; 47 Laura Wickenden; 48 (bottom) The Bridgeman Art Library; 50–51 Images Colour Library; 52 Camera Press; 53 Henry Arden; 56 Laura Wickenden; 62 Robert Harding Picture Library; 64 Laura Wickenden; 66 Laura Wickenden; 67 Henry Arden; 68–69 Science Photo Library; 70 Laura Wickenden; 73 (bottom) Laura Wickenden; 74–75 Laura Wickenden; 76–77 Science Photo Library; 84 Marshall Editions; 85–86 Science Photo Library; 88 Henry Arden; 93 The Stock Market; 103 (bottom) Henry Arden; 121 Henry Arden; 123 (left) Science Photo Library (right) The Stock Market; 125 Henry Arden; 129 Henry Arden; 137 Tony Latham; 140–142 Henry Arden; 148 Henry Arden; 149 (left) Henry Arden; 151 Laura Wickenden; 160 Science Photo Library; 161 Laura Wickenden; 165 Laura Wickenden; 167 Henry Arden; 169 Henry Arden